THE
INSPIRED
Therapist

MY INNER JOURNEY FROM WANNABE TO HEALER

by Howard Scott Warshaw, MA, ME, LMFT

The Silicon Valley Therapist

"Passion with a balanced perspective."

California License Number: MFT 52529

Published By: SCOTT WEST Productions

Book Design By: TommyOwenDesign.com

ISBN #: 978-0-9862186-2-0

Version 2.0

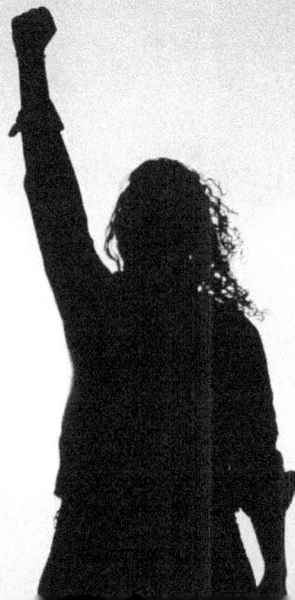

Dedication

TO SHERRI, MY WIFE,
WHO PROVES MIRACLES
ARE POSSIBLE WHEN WE'RE
INSPIRED BY HOPE AND DESIRE.

Table of Contents

Passion ☯ Perspective

"To sense the client's world as if it were your own, but without ever losing the 'as if' quality – this is empathy and this seems essential to therapy."

Carl Rogers

"Every experience, no matter how bad it seems, holds within it a blessing of some kind. The goal is to find it."

Buddha

THE POWER OF PERSPECTIVE

Do you remember a puzzle you couldn't solve? That was a difficult problem. Then you received the solution and suddenly the problem became easy. The puzzle changed from impossible to simple yet the puzzle never changed... you did! You came upon a different way to look at the problem which made it easy to solve. You shifted your point of view and found a new approach.

Locking ourselves into limited perspectives shrinks the world. When we are free to shift our perspective and adopt different points of view, more solutions become available to us. We become better able to find productive alternatives when challenges come our way.

We become more effective problem solvers when we work less on our problems and more on ourselves.

WELCOME TO PSY-MART

I'm shopping for a theory. This is my current priority as a student/trainee hurtling toward graduation and internship. I need a therapeutic identity to facilitate the process. So, I head down to Psy-Mart (Costco for psychotherapists), grab a cart and start browsing. There's DBT, EFT, CBT, EVT, DDP, etc. So many TLAs (Three Letter Acronyms). Between the BBS, my GPA and my CPA, my EKG needs some TLC if I'm ever to be an MFT. OMG!

Every theory is another perspective. So different yet so similar, and they all have their TLAs. There's Psychodynamic (a seed was planted in your head), then there's Behavioral (all around you seeds are flying at your head), and then there's Humanistic (forget about the seeds, I love your head). There's Systemic (it takes many heads to truly plant a seed), and then there's the ever present Existential (I'm all alone, I'm going to die, there's no point and I'm responsible) which may sound bleak but it has the best jokes.

Sometimes I learn a lot from TLAs. For instance, I like CBT but I'm not crazy about Behavioral in general. There is just something about the world of pure stimulus/response that strips me of my creative individuality and I don't like it. However, I think the Cognitive aspect is fantastic because I'm totally mental. I figure I'll just take the B out of CBT and there will be my perfect theory, and interestingly that turns out to be true. When I remove the 'B' I'm left with CT (Counter Transference). This makes me look at why I react as I do to the Behavioral models and I think, "Oh yeah, Adlerian strivings to overcome lack of acknowledgement in my past made me sensitive to perceived depersonalization. I will do my best to remain mindful of this, particularly when treating clients with Narcissistic issues." Sometimes TLA's can inform us.

I enjoy using humor, but occasionally I use it to mask my resistance. I experience pushback when selecting a theory. I feel by selecting one I'm denying all the others. Systemic seems natural to me as a former engineer and cognitive makes so much sense. The precepts of existentialism were undeniable facts to me from a very young age and Buddhism is similarly intuitive to me. I believe psychodynamic theory is a necessary but not sufficient approach and the research clearly demonstrates they all need a humanistic component to succeed. In my dreams, I seamlessly integrate all theories and eliminate the need for a choice, but this a dream. Instead I'm taking time and care, looking around to find the best theoretical fit for me. But what if I make the wrong choice?

Two soothing thoughts come to mind. The first is simply realizing this is not the last choice. I can always switch theories as time, knowledge and practice dictate. The second thought is something I heard from a wise colleague, "Forget about making the right choice. There is no wrong choice." One aspect of becoming a therapist is accepting a world rife with opportunities to second guess myself. The best way to avoid it: just don't do it.

As I think about selecting a theory, I value every opportunity to gain perspective and insight which ultimately helps me serve my clients. I can choose to see this as obsessing over making perfect choices, but I prefer to reframe it as simply being a smart shopper.

WISDOM

Wisdom is a commodity, mined from the ore of our mistakes. We are each of us sitting on the mother lode.

Some say those who do not learn from their mistakes are doomed to repeat them. But those who do learn from mistakes are now in a position to go forward and make new ones… hopefully!

I used to fear making mistakes. Consequently I approached any new endeavor with great caution and reserve. Too much looking and not enough leaping. Now when I set out to learn something new I jump in. I try to make as many mistakes as I can as quickly as possible.

I stopped trying to avoid mistakes and simply focused on not repeating them. Ironically, the further I get from perfect the more my performance improves.

Passion ☯ Perspective

"Living with integrity means:
Not settling for less than what you
know you deserve in your relationships.
Asking for what you want and need
from others. Speaking your truth,
even though it might create conflict or
tension. Behaving in ways that are in
harmony with your personal values.
Making choices based on what you
believe, and not what others believe."

Barbara De Angelis

FUNDAMENTAL QUESTIONS
OF PERSONALITY

There are simple questions whose answers define us. I call these Fundamental Questions of Personality. One of my favorites is: "Would you rather be right or kind?"

Preferring "right" may indicate a more objective or removed stance. A perspective that is independent of circumstance and justifiable.

Preferring "kind" can indicate a more relational or connected stance. A more accepting and less judgmental point of view.

Each has its strengths and weaknesses. Each has its place and time.

Yet each of us tends to lean a bit more toward one than the other. Some of us lean a lot! And some people simply need to be one or the other.

One thing I wonder about the people who need to be right... Was it ever OK to just be them?

THE CHANGE

Change. Some say it's the only constant. As inevitable as death and taxes. I believe becoming a therapist is all about change, and change is all about choices; the ones you make and the ones you don't. Choice is the difference between changing and evolving. The most important question to answer is this: "What do I want to do?"

For many years and entire careers I chose to avoid that question by doing what I could do, what seemed practical to do and what I thought I ought to do. This is likely why I kept changing careers. At one point my heart actually got a word in edgewise and helped my head acknowledge what the rest of me always knew, I want to be a therapist. Great! Choice made. Bring on the change. I set my sights on the MFT path and started marching forward.

Then one day, right in the middle of my matriculation, a new acronym came to town, LPCC (Latest Professional Credential Conundrum). Are you kidding me? I finally commit to a degree and it turns out I'm taking the wrong classes? I was frustrated. The universe wasn't cooperating. Then I got over myself and realized two things. First, this is simply the nature of growth. Each choice invites change and each change poses new choices, so roll with it or get rolled by it. Second, becoming a therapist is not so much a thing to do but rather a way to be. As a recovering "do" person, I need a new approach since my path of choice is a changing one.

Recently I read a book which focused on the difference between transition and transformation. It defined transition as meeting some external criteria whereas transformation meant undergoing fundamental internal change. For example, when the BBS taps you on both shoulders with the license and dubs you "Therapist," this is a transition. However, overcoming self-doubt and inexperience so you can sit in the room with clients and truly believe you can be of service, that's a transformation. Transition is about doing, transformation is about being.

I started to think of getting credentials (licenses, certifications) as a transition. I also saw gaining expertise as a transformation. In the world of licensing boards, credentials are mandatory but expertise is optional. As proof, I invite you to consider your fellow licensed drivers.

Remembering that getting credentials and gaining expertise are two separate tasks actually helps me. Rather than feeling like a burden, it keeps me mindful. The track to licensure is intensely focused on rules and structure. It's easy to get so buried under the onslaught of BBS regulations and paperwork that clinical work with clients becomes that thing I do between case notes, intakes, supervision and studying. I experience mantra-shift and start to think: To be a therapist, I only need to be licensed.

That's when mindfulness comes in. I think of credentials *and* expertise. It helps me value my clinical time and remember that in order to be the therapist I want to be, I must remain vigilant, present and attend to both.

On second thought, maybe it's not so important to answer the question: "What do I want to do?" Perhaps it's wiser to choose to change the question to: "How am I and how shall I be?" And that's a choice I don't want to change.

PASSION WITH A BALANCED PERSPECTIVE

"Passion with a Balanced Perspective" is my life philosophy (or at least the goal I strive for).

Passion is the source of tremendous energy. There are many things about which I am very passionate. Being a psychotherapist is chief among them. I have been fortunate to enjoy many different careers, each with its own particular intrigue and perspective. Psychotherapy draws on all the others. It brings my entire past to life and lets me reach more types of people in deeper ways.

A Balanced Perspective sustains the energy. Without balance I can simply burn brightly until I burn out. Balance brings focus and direction to the energy. Balance helps me choose where to spend the energy and when to shift.

Passion creates the fire. Balance creates the lamp. This is very useful when exploring dark and unfamiliar places, as therapists frequently do.

As a therapist I inspire clients to seek passion with a balanced perspective. Then they're empowered to pursue their own journey.

Passion ☯ Perspective

"The body is trying to say
what the mouth can't say."

Virginia Satir

"People hate as they love,
unreasonably."

William Makepeace Thackeray

"You can avoid reality, but you
cannot avoid the consequences
of avoiding reality."

Ayn Rand

SOME WORDS ON NON-VERBAL COMMUNICATION

We teach others how to treat us by the way we treat ourselves. Talk is cheap! Showing is more powerful than telling.

The old adage "do as I say, not as I do" is absurd. You might as well say "I'm a hypocrite." Our choices (demonstrated through our actions) reveal our true desires and beliefs.

When people are mistreating me, it's worthwhile to take a break from blaming them and really examine how I've been acting. I may want people to treat me more respectfully, but am I too self-effacing or deprecating? I may want you to take me more seriously, but have I been acting out inappropriately?

As a therapist, what I say goes hand-in-hand with what I'm modeling… or it doesn't. Self-care, healthy boundaries and being authentic are solid recommendations for clients. But do I model them as well? Clients can see and feel if I am.

What I tell clients is one thing, but how I act is the non-verbal communication which demonstrates my genuine priorities and convictions. This is the more powerful lesson that those around me will take to heart.

In the room, just as in life, my actions speak louder than my words. That's why it's so important for me to do as I recommend!

THERAPEUTIC PERSPECTIVES

One question plagues me as I march toward licensure: What makes a good therapist? Is it insight? Outcome? Empathy? Diagnostic accuracy? Minimum counter transference? Maximum income? I think the answer lies in perspective. I think about perspective a lot.

Perspective is fun to play with, particularly when it shows us how we limit ourselves. Is the glass half empty or half full? Perhaps the glass is too large. As we shift perspectives we open new doors, creating new sources of light. Perspective is also the key to problem solving. There are no hard or easy problems, there are simply helpful and unhelpful perspectives. We solve problems by adopting a useful perspective for the situation. For example: Logic Puzzles.

Remember a logic puzzle you couldn't solve? It seemed like a really tough puzzle. Then you learned the solution and suddenly it was an easy puzzle. But the puzzle never changed, you did. You incorporated a new perspective and that changed everything.

In my perspective on therapy, each modality represents another perspective on working with a client. I've heard there are over 200 recognized therapeutic modalities, and millions of unique potential clients. That's a lot of combinations, so I use a systemic construct (perspective) called "the healing trinity" to hold it in my head.

The healing trinity consists of The Client, The Modality and The Therapist. I believe for every Client there is an optimal Modality and a Therapist who can skillfully apply this modality while building effective rapport with this client. When the three components are well matched they achieve a beautiful synergy called "therapeutic progress," which is something I have learned not to define specifically but, if you'll pardon my judgment, it's a good thing. The healing trinity is my perspective for framing a concept of being a good therapist. First, let's define the spectrum.

At one end is the ultimate therapist: the Modal Goddess. She connects instantly and deeply with everyone she meets and applies every modality flawlessly. At the other end of the spectrum is the worst possible therapist: the Lucky Schnook. This is a guy so off-putting he needed over two thousand clients to make his hours because no one would see him twice, then he lucky-guessed his way through the exams. Now he is licensed but clueless. These are hypothetical extremes, of course, but hypothesis is an essential part of life. Can you imagine a world with no hypothetical situations?

Most of us lay somewhere in between the Lucky Schnook and the Modal Goddess. Exactly where depends on our current perspective. As I shift perspective toward the Modal Goddess I'm improving. There are two components of the trinity I can control, the modality and the therapist. Every time I achieve competency in a new modality or improve my skills in one I already practice, I'm taking a step toward the Modal Goddess. Each time I uncover a new source of counter transference and learn to observe it, each time I increase my capacity for acceptance and each time I improve my holding capacity or increase inner peace, I'm getting closer still.

Then there's the client. The starting point. The component I don't control. I feel respect is the key. I take a step toward the Modal Goddess by remembering the client is the one with the answers if only I can hear them clearly. I endeavor to appreciate my client as I would Leonardo DaVinci or Albert Einstein. I do this by reminding myself of one basic truth: everyone is the genius of their own perspective.

THE "MONDAY" REFRAME

A lot of people hate Mondays. At times I have felt this way too. Consider this…

Monday's are only about 14% of your life (~14.2857% for the more retentive among us). When you wake up on any given day you are a 6-to-1 favorite to avoid it! Those are pretty good odds.

What about Mondays when you don't have to go to work or school? Are those better Mondays? When you add the fact most 3-day weekends include Monday and every week long vacation includes a Monday, that's still quite a few Mondays back in the win column.

And after all, is it really Monday you hate? Or is it what you must do on Monday? And why do you hate this thing so much that you feel the need to transfer your ire on to an innocent day of the week? In Israel, the weekend is Friday and Saturday. I wonder if they hate Sunday?

I've noticed two periods in my life when I was consistently happy on Monday: Long ago when I was at Atari creating some of the first video games and the last several years since I've become a psycho-therapist. I like Monday because I love what I'm doing.

So when Monday hurts a bit, take heart in the knowledge that it's probably not Monday that irks you, it's your life. This is great news, because it's so much easier to change your life than it is to change the week!

Passion ☯ Perspective

"Between stimulus and response, there is a space. In that space lies our freedom and power to choose our response. In our response lies our growth and freedom."

Victor Frankl

"Where there is great love, there are always miracles."

Willa Cather

FORGIVENESS

Every time I forgive someone, I'm giving a tremendous gift... to myself!

Traditionally we see forgiveness as something we give to others. But I believe, if we are wise, forgiveness is something we take for ourselves. Here's why:

When we feel slighted or wronged by someone we can invest a lot of energy into the situation. We look for confederates to validate how we were wronged. We may plot revenge. We may seek to broadcast the incident in order to "correct" their reputation. Most importantly, though, we hang on to it. We start investing energy in taking offense and being upset. How long we continue is up to us.

Forgiveness is frequently misunderstood in this context. Forgiveness is not condoning or ratifying what they did. Forgiveness is the act of releasing myself from having to waste fresh energy and thoughts on a past I didn't create and certainly cannot change.

When I get truly upset, my body produces consequences that deplete my resources and diminish my immune system, rendering me more vulnerable to illness. I can literally worry myself sick.

Forgiveness gives me permission to move forward with my life rather than remain stuck in a negative place created by someone else. Many wise people suggest unkind acts are really an expression of the perpetrator's pain or fear, the victim just happens to be there at the time. In this view, forgiveness is releasing the issues of others and getting back on my own path.

Forgiveness doesn't mean I'm OK with what you did. It means I'm letting your problems remain yours and I'm returning my focus to my own goals.

For me, this is a precious gift indeed!

MIRROR, MIRROR

I'm starting to realize becoming a psychotherapist is very much about image.

My journey toward licensure is well under way now. I have a primary theory or two, my classes are finished, academic requirements are met, hours are accumulating and after a year of seeing clients I'm turning the corner and feeling like I belong in the room. I'm peri-therapausal.

One of my favorite things about becoming a therapist is the teachers: supervisors, professors, mentors, colleagues, anyone from whom I may learn (which, when I'm on my game, is basically everyone). One of my favorite teachers speaks about the importance of metaphor. She challenges me to find a metaphor for how I imagine practicing therapy. So I head back to PsyMart and start browsing the therapeutic self-image isles to see what's on sale. I find myself buying into the Mirror Repairman kit whose theme is: "Mirror Repairmen help people perceive themselves more clearly." I can see myself wearing the little tool belt full of techniques and cute therapist hat, going to work and leaving a happier and higher functioning world in my wake. The image fits, the price is right and Halloween is here.

I'm strolling toward checkout with a satisfied air, chanting along with the singing bowls being piped in over the loudspeakers, when something in the clearance bin catches my eye.

"Every block of stone has a statue inside and it's the task of the sculptor to discover it." — Michelangelo. OMG! This quote is really calling to me. The answer lies inside you. I help my client discover their statue. What a beautiful and powerful image. Not only is it an amazing metaphor but it's marked down 70%! Then I notice another therapist eyeing it. In a flash I leave my feet, diving into the bin and securing my prize. That was close. After dealing with the ethical dilemma of having left the Mirror Repairman set at the bottom of the bin, I press on toward checkout.

Just as I'm approaching the register I notice a little point-of-purchase display. There I see: "Art is not truth. Art is a lie which makes us realize truth." — Pablo Picasso. Hmmm, now that's an interesting metaphor. It's pithy and dramatic and fits a different part of my image. At times we prescribe the symptom or tell a parallel story about another "client" or "couple." We tell the lie intended to help our client realize their truth. I like the way this speaks to the client's realization rather than my work of discovery. I can also hear my teacher saying "You shouldn't work harder than your client."

Next to Picasso I see another gem by Michelangelo, "I saw the angel in the marble and carved until I set him free." I like the idea of setting the angel free, but the carving is a little too directive for me. My head is spinning with all these designer metaphors, each makes an important point and no one is enough. I decide to just go home and make my own.

At home I sit down with my conceptual sewing machine, stitching up a composite image. Between Michelangelo and Picasso I realize the content of my desired metaphor for practicing therapy. The image I'm seeking reflects my desire to help clients realize and recognize within themselves the person they'd prefer to be, then aid them in allowing this person to emerge into presence and being. It's not really a sculptor, it's kind of a tour guide. It's a work in progress.

Perhaps *I'm* the statue in the stone, continually cutting away the parts that blind me from discovering the therapist within me. One challenge of becoming a therapist is to weather constant introspection and change. I'll keep working on my ultimate metaphor and if I never get there that's fine too. I can always go back into mirror repair.

CAN PEOPLE CHANGE?

Do you believe people can change? Can people actually become different in their beliefs and inclinations?

This is a Fundamental Question of Personality.

Some believe that somewhere between the ages of 5 and 10 we lock in a personality and that's it. You are who you will ever be.

There are others who believe change is not only possible but inevitable. That we are not the same person from moment to moment, let alone decade to decade.

Some say change happens unconsciously, others feel they are always available for reconstruction but only when the need or desire strikes.

There are many variations on the theme, but at the end of the day there is little confusion about it. When it comes to the issue of fundamental change, there are two kinds of people: Those who say it's possible and those who say it's not.

There may be two kinds of people but there are all kinds of psychotherapists, each with their own approach, theoretical orientation, style, outlook and counter-transference. No two are the same. But they all share one thing in common: Every psychotherapist takes it as basic truth that people are able to change. Certainly there are people who don't or won't change, people who refuse or resist change… but every therapist maintains that anyone is capable of change.

And it cannot possibly be otherwise. Because the moment a therapist stops believing people can change, they are no longer a therapist…

They have become a hypocrite.

Passion ☯ Perspective

"Every human being's essential
nature is perfect and faultless, but
after years of immersion in the world
we easily forget our roots and take on
a counterfeit nature."

Lao-Tzu, (6th century BCE)

"Do not let the behavior of others
destroy your inner peace."

Dalai Lama

CUPID'S ONGOING CHALLENGE

The people we love do things that change us. Our vulnerability gives them this power.

When I open my feelings to you in a loving relationship, things you do affect me. When the effect is profound, I change. Similarly, some things I do change you. Throughout this process we are each becoming different people because of the closeness we share.

As long as we both grow and change, we are constantly creating a new relationship. If we stagnate then nothing changes… except time passing, which creates its own pressures.

Either way, it changes how our love is. What does loving each other mean now?

I believe when we first meet someone we don't fall in love with them, we merely begin loving them. Then, if we choose to, we commit to keep re-finding a new love to share.

Cupid's job is not an easy one. Love is a moving target.

THE ORALS STAGE

I have Oral Exams next week (the developmental challenge for my current stage of becoming a therapist). After years of working, studying, paying and hundreds of clinical hours I am now facing the last hurdle in my quest for internship. If I pass, I need only sustain a pulse for a few months and I'm there. That will feel good. Much better than I'm feeling right now.

I wish it was my licensure exam, I picture that as being much easier and less anxiety producing. Although I remember preparing for my qualifying written exam a year ago and thinking I'd much rather be taking my oral exam since that will probably be much easier and less anxiety producing. So, in an effort to reduce the stress I'm studying for the exam. Or rather, I should be.

Instead I'm writing this column. Am I resisting or drifting? Maybe I'm blocked. Should I fight the blockage and study on, accept the blockage and let it go or explore the blockage and work my way through it. Which is more productive? I'm aware of the moment but not entirely in it. I am, however, watching it very closely so I won't miss anything… except the experience.

I realize the choices I make now during these early stages of my therapeutic development will establish patterns for my future behavior. I can shift to the future: Will they be adaptive or maladaptive? I can shift to the past: How did I deal with the challenges of earlier stages? Or I can choose to return to the present: Why am I still not studying? Aha, I caught myself wandering.

Amid this internal debate, I see I'm focused on the present but not being present. In chatting most enjoyably with myself, I'm merely distracting-from rather than being-in the moment. How can I stop talking about being here and just be here? Hmmm, let's discuss that.

But discussion is not the answer, experience is. During case presentations I talk about corrective *experiences*, not corrective *discussions*. I should talk with myself about how to be more experiential. No, I should just be, just be, just be…

It occurs to me amidst my tangential reverie that what I'm being in the current moment is a person who is still not studying. It's the test! That damn test is so anxietizing. It's an absurd exception to what really has been a wonderful curriculum, and the format is… OMG! I'm Counter-Transferred! I'm experiencing Academic Counter-Transference. I need exam therapy, STAT! I schedule an emergency session. My therapist informs me that "Academic Counter-Transference" is a pretty rare condition and this is more likely a case of just drifting a little. She recommends I simply relax and take the test. She's right.

OK, so my mind is wandering a bit. This also happens in the room. There I know when I catch myself wandering it's a signal something is going on right here right now. I can acknowledge it, own it and rejoin the experience, possibly with a new awareness. Maybe that's a good lesson. When I notice I'm drifting, follow the departure rather than attack it. I know the material for my oral exam, but I'm afraid pieces might disappear during the test inviting catastrophe. That fear distracts me. But I have a choice. If I forget something on the test I can come back to it with curiosity rather than freeze in panic or self-judgment. I don't have to "catch" myself wandering, instead I can "find" myself wandering. I guess I have been studying for orals after all.

NORMALCY

"Every advance in civilization has been denounced as unnatural while it was recent." Bertrand Russell, (1872-1970)

And it was! By definition, change is always abnormal.

As a therapist, one question I hear a lot is "What's normal?" The best definition of normal that I've encountered so far is: Normal is what you're used to. Therefore, anything you are not used to will seem abnormal or unnatural.

We treat normal like some universal standard when actually it's a very individual quality. We each have our own normal. Any time someone wants to make a change, the first step is becoming abnormal. Over time, if the deviation remains present and consistent, the new way becomes typical and is no longer judged abnormal. At this point, "normal" has been reset and change has occurred.

Dissatisfaction motivates desire for change which leads to deviation from normal. Repeated deviance begets a new consistency which, if maintained, ultimately creates a new "normal."

Some say normal leads to right angles and wrong turns.

My favorite definition of "normal" came from an old golfing buddy who used to say, "Normal people are people you just don't know very well."

Passion ☯ Perspective

"Don't work on the client. We do our work which lets them do theirs."

Maria Klein, MFT

"And the day came when the desire to stay the same was more painful than the risk to evolve."

Unknown

VISUALIZATION:
SUBLIME OR RIDICULOUS

Some people give Visualization a bad rap. They say the idea of achieving something by merely picturing it is childish fantasy. Wishful thinking not based in reality. And if that's all there was to visualization, they'd be right.

But that's not all there is to visualization.

Visualization is a tool. And like any tool, its power rests entirely in the skill of its user.

But it's even more than that! Visualization is a mechanism. When used properly, Visualization ignites a fuse… activating me toward achieving my goals.

Visualization isn't about conjuring a whim. Visualization is about defining my future. Designing my destination. Specifically. Thoroughly. With Crystalline Clarity.

This brings my goal into incredibly sharp focus. What's at the root of almost every success story ever told? Clear identifiable goals!

Now I know how to direct my energy. As I contemplate options, I can answer the question: "Does this move me closer to my goal or not?" Goodbye analysis paralysis!

Visualization helps me set my intention, which helps me focus my energies, which enables me to bring my full potential to bear on tasks. And that's when goals are achieved!

THE DUALITY OF CLOSURE

Finally, oral exams are a thing of the passed and I've satisfied all my graduation requirements. Having met the challenge of this developmental stage I'm ready to close the door on another chapter of my psychotherapeutic odyssey. Time to pop the corks and engage in some serious self-care. Bring on the serenity!

But when one door closes another one opens, and sometimes that next door buries me in an avalanche of new To-Do's. The prospect of internship (with the duties, responsibilities and all the hours thereto appertaining) looms large before me. It all seems so confrontational. After such a long climb I've only reached the bottom of an even longer staircase. Where's the afterglow?

When I take a moment to stop and reflect, things do look pretty good. I passed my final qualifying exam and survived my rite of passage. This boosted my confidence and helped my therapeutic self-image substantially. I can see myself making the crucial transition from wondering if I can be a therapist to knowing I will be a therapist, which feels wonderful. And just the other day I had back-to-back sessions in which clients achieved long sought-after breakthroughs. Ah, there's the glow. I'm smoking big Freudian cigars.

But you know how it goes. The very next morning I experience a client who seems to have misplaced all their progress. I'm reminded that I have groups to plan and run, a full client load, scheduling conflicts to resolve, case documentation due, an intake backlog and BOOM! The cigar explodes right in my face (the cigar is, of course, just a cigar). Suddenly the prospect of maintaining a pulse until graduation sounds like… well, a lot more than autonomic functioning.

But that's OK. I can go forward doing all I'm doing and taking on more. That's what I signed up for. It just bothers me that there's no big pop here. Something's missing. I expected to feel more… something.

I guess anticipated feelings are tricky things. They don't always show up on schedule. Perhaps it's better to let the feelings flow and just welcome them as they arrive rather than sending out invitations and expecting RSVP's. That whole mindfulness/presence thing again. I've learned it so many times and I'm still learning it. I'm getting better at being present with clients; having less expectation of progress and accepting they'll proceed at their own pace. It's harder to let go of my expectations for me however, trying to control my own pace. Trying to match my own ideas of how I'm supposed to be or feel as I move forward in my training. It also makes me a bit self-conscious. I worry about being the only psychotherapy intern with control issues. But who am I kidding? Do I think no one will notice? Hanging out with a bunch of therapists is like going to an emotional nude beach. On the one hand it's a silly place for the excessively self-conscious, and on the other hand my fellow sun lovers are very accepting so there's really nothing to fear. And hopefully on the other hand is a generous dollop of sun block.

My point is I face three choices when a milestone is reached: I can look longingly back on where I've been (regress), I can tremble before the onslaught of new challenges (stagnate), or I can try to remain accepting of where I am and move forward with mindful awareness.

One door closes and another opens. Reframe 1: When one obligation is over, another steps right in to fill the void. Reframe 2: With each challenge met, a new plateau of opportunity presents itself. Sure, it sounds nicer in the second framing. But sometimes the fear of more substantial obstacles finds me desperately trying to get back through the door I just closed. In fact, I can be so busy banging on that door I miss the chance to savor the beautiful new view created as the next door gently blows open. In other words: when a door closes on a chapter of your life, don't knock it.

THE QUESTION MARK OF LIFE

During my graduation ceremony, bedecked in pomp and circumstance on a beautifully manicured plush green lawn, it suddenly struck me: While I was supposed to be having a time stopping moment, the rest of the world kept right on moving. Clocks kept ticking, cars kept rolling. The big transition was in my head only, and even that felt a bit blurry.

As a writer I am keenly aware that punctuation is critical. It conveys timing, delineates concepts and alters meaning. Without punctuation one idea simply runs into the next. Without punctuation we lose clarity, pace and dramatic impact.

There are monumental moments in life. The final step of one arduous journey or the very first step of another. Moments so large it seems time itself should stop for a breath and a nod, but of course it does not. Life's continuity is magnificent but it also feels disappointing at times. This torrential momentum renders some of my significant moments anti-climactic.

The cure is releasing any expectation of breaks and literally go with the flow. Embrace continuity rather than oppose it. Yet there is something appealing about stopping to smell the roses, counting our chickens and eating our ice cream before it melts. I miss the commas, the exclamation points and of course… the elipses.

But alas, there is no punctuation in life. Period!

Passion ☯ Perspective

Therapists cannot force people
to change, we can only invite them.
As we learn to make nicer invitations,
we start throwing better parties.

The healing power of Art lies in
its ability to give you control in
a world with no rules!

RESPONSIBILITY

Responsibility is not about accepting blame. Responsibility is about recognizing that the power to change things around me rests solely in my ability to change myself.

After all, I'm the only person I can change. This thought leaves some people feeling disempowered. How can I have impact if I can't change others?

The relief rests in one fact: We live in a relational world. We are affected by our interactions with others. When the people around me change, I adapt. This constitutes a change for me.

Which means whenever I change, I create change for others. I have changed their world and they adapt, which changes them.

I can withdraw from others or engage them. I can seek to inhibit others or find ways to inspire them. The choice of direction is mine. The choice of reaction is theirs. I cannot control the implications of this change, but those implications are no less awesome.

When I change myself… when I truly shift my perspective on how to approach life… I am literally changing the world!

"INTERN-ALIZED"

"To be is to do." Socrates
"To do is to be." Sartre
"Do be do be do." Sinatra

More on these three quotes in a moment.

As of this writing I am no longer a Trainee. I have made the leap to Associate MFT or Intern. This is a purely titular transition of course (based solely on completing my Master's degree) and does not warrant any actual change on my part. Nonetheless it does invite reflection. Has anything really changed since beginning this journey nearly four years ago?

Back then I envisioned practicing therapy as sitting in a comfy chair doling out life-altering insights to idealized clients who receive them with sincere gratitude in a spirit of bonhomie followed immediately by a generous check. Now, as my clinical hours approach four figures I'm finding this is not my typical experience in the room. I'm not *working on* clients so much as *being with* clients. Instead of a convivial and analytically removed experience I'm engaging my clients by building intimate connections, or at least holding open the possibility. This not only serves my clients but also comes back to me in so many marvelous growth lessons. The reality is fulfilling rather than disillusioning. I feel truly blessed. Even more so since the fantasy was so sweet!

Another realization I've gained from seeing clients is that holding therapeutic space for a person is a difficult task. Being with a distressed client without turning off, without judging, without drifting, staying present and connected while sitting in a place of empathy is a tough thing to do. One challenge of therapy is earnestly facing the fact that being a healer means regularly confronting real pain, distress and damage. "Self-care" sounds trite in introductory seminars but the more I learn the more this concept deepens for me.

Then there's the unconscious facet of my transformation. I had a dream a few weeks ago in which I met a person who became angry with me upon learning I was becoming a therapist. He told me, "I don't like that you're becoming a therapist. My wife wants us to go to marriage counseling. You therapists think you know people, but you don't know #%@&! You sure as hell don't know anything about me!"

So my dream response was, "I know one thing about you. I know you really don't like my becoming a therapist. This shows me you get pretty upset over things that have nothing to do with you. Maybe you expect people around you to support you or make you feel good about yourself. This is a lot to put on others, particularly when it's a covert demand. And the one person you likely hold most responsible for supplying this good feeling is your partner, which isn't automatically bad for your relationship. You might have a partner who lacks self-confidence, is highly dependent and needs help defining goals and behavioral norms. That could be very symbiotic. On the other hand if your partner is an independent person who expects you to support them just as they support you, then that might become a source of tension in your relationship. It could go either way I suppose. But didn't you just say she wants to try couples counseling? Hmmm, perhaps that's a second thing I know about you." And I woke up smiling.

I smiled because this dream simply made me feel I'd learned a lot about clinical thinking in the last few years, and that is a very nice feeling for me.

Upon reflection, the three opening quotes reflect some key lessons for me in becoming a therapist. As a writer, filmmaker and high tech denizen for decades I was all about doing. Now I have come to believe that therapy is all about being. Being is more attuned than doing. My main challenge as an Intern is relaxing into being (no small task for a recovering doer). These three quotes guide me in this pursuit. Socrates affirms my goals, Sartre warns me of my habits, and Sinatra alludes lyrically to my ongoing "Intern-al" struggle.

HOW TO PACK FOR TIME TRAVEL

Ever run into an old acquaintance and start reminiscing? They tell you a story and you recall it instantly, but you also realize that until this moment you'd completely forgotten it. Possibly lost forever if my old friend doesn't rekindle the memory. We don't realize this until we compare notes with others. When it does happen it briefly opens a window into ourselves. If you care to, take a look.

We take what we need from any moment, but we don't take all there is... or was. We make choices as to what we carry forward and what we leave behind. How do we decide? The choices we make say a great deal about who we are. They show us what we are seeking as we venture on through life. When my old friend reminds me of a choice I made, it gives me the chance to explore.

This process of selecting which memories to carry is very much like packing for a long trip. I focus on the things I believe will best serve me in my travels.

I pack very carefully for the journey into my future, because what I pack determines where I'm heading.

Passion ☯ Perspective

"You never change things by fighting the existing reality. To change something, build a new model that makes the existing model obsolete."

Buckminster Fuller

"Great spirits have always encountered violent opposition from mediocre minds."

Albert Einstein

THE STORM & THE DESERT

At times I find it interesting to view anxiety as a storm and depression as a desert. This clarifies goals.

With anxiety I want to calm the storm. With depression I want to find the oasis.

In the storm, the way to calm is to speak a fundamental undeniable truth. When heard, this dissipates the turbulence and allows for a place of quiet contemplation.

In the desert, a shower of accurate appreciation and empathy combined with gratitude can create an oasis. This offers a destination amidst the arid dunes.

When the storm and desert come into balance, the result is fertile land.

THERAPIST IN THE ROOM!

Empathy is a funny thing. In fact yesterday it made my personal therapist hysterical. I was sharing my challenges in working with a particularly vexing client when suddenly an empathetic thought struck me, "This was probably what I was like in *our* first sessions." We took a short break as she gasped for air while convulsing with laughter. Therapeutic karma? Who knows? Unique moments arise when therapists become clients.

Like the time my therapist gave me the same advice I had given to a client earlier that same day. I mean she used the exact same phrase, word for word. Neither of us had ever said it before. This led to self-questioning and a counter transference witch hunt. Fortunately my therapist happened to be there at the time.

But what was up with that?! Was I speaking to myself rather than my client? I must admit there are times in the room when I cast a pearl and as I hear myself say it I think, "That's a pretty good idea, I should take that advice myself." I guess we are who we treat.

I certainly am… at least from one point of view. I find I'm very different in the room from client to client (my therapist says she's the same way, she just can't model it for me). On a good day I'll frame this as being flexible, engaged and attuned to my client's needs. I meet them where they are and stay present in that place with them. On a tough day I might wonder if I'm just being erratic. Perhaps it comes down to my motivation.

As a therapist I try to give my client what they need. There are, however, many shades of "what my client needs." There's what they say they need, what I think they need, what they think I want to hear them need, what I need for myself but project onto them… and somewhere amidst all this is what my client actually needs. This can coincide with any of the above or be a whole other thing entirely. Contemplating client needs can lead to the need for aspirin.

All this is simplified by one of the best things I've learned in my journey: Being authentic and modeling congruency. It's not only good practice, it also saves a lot of mental energy. I simply follow Socrates' ancient dictum "Know Thyself," then live what I've learned. However, this raises another question: If I'm being so authentic, why am I so different from client to client? It seems a bit contradictory. The answer is found in another great thing I've learned along the way: Don't get bogged down in content, concentrate on process. What I'm trying to do is connect authentically with each client, that's my process. It's the same in each case but it looks different from client to client because every client is unique. It's just like an interpreter at the United Nations. They sound different when sharing a message in several different languages but the process is the same in each case: communication.

I have a lot of questions. As a registered intern with over half my hours I'm tempted to think I should have more answers by now. But like they say: Every answer spawns ten more questions. One that keeps coming back to me in different forms is this: What is therapy like for my clients? Are they getting something positive? Are they growing and moving forward? I always picture experienced therapists as being past these issues but I'm not that experienced yet (and some experienced therapists tell me I never will be).

As empathetic as I may be I still cannot directly experience my client's experience. However, as a therapist in therapy, I do get a special kind of validation. I can appreciate my therapeutic experience; the comforts, the struggles and the growth. I understand that the particulars of my therapy are different from everyone else's, but the process is still the same. This reaffirms my sense of value about what I offer my clients, and on the occasional tough day it buoys me.

WHAT MAKES A GOOD COUPLE?

Individuals come to therapy to make a change. Couples come to therapy to make their partner change (hopefully before changing partners). At least that's how it starts.

Everyone is the genius of their own perspective. We know how things should be in our world, and we tend to view our partner's behavior through this lens. In difficult times, it's clear to me how my partner needs to change in order to get things back on track. Of course, my partner has the same helpful advice for me.

We rarely assess our own behavior through our partner's eyes. After all, I'm not the genius of *their* perspective. Nonetheless we are two trains in the same tunnel and unless we coordinate our expectations there's going to be a crash. Couple's therapy is about avoiding the collision or repairing and rerouting afterward.

How do you know when it works? The couple knows… when they reassess their relationship. A couple is in good shape when each partner feels they're getting the best of the bargain.

UNIQUE LIKE ME

We are all pretty clear on the fact that everyone is unique. We are all different in some way or another. We like different styles and surroundings. Our taste in movies and books varies a great deal. And of course there's that whole thing about horse races...

But we also expect others, on a fundamental level, to think like us. To have the same basic reactions and assessments... and we're frequently flummoxed when they don't.

Everyone is unique yet we still expect others to see things as we do. It makes for limitless comedy and limiting presumptions.

Passion ☯ Perspective

"Sometimes you win,
sometimes you learn."

Robert Kiyosaki

"You can tell whether a man is clever by
his answers. You can tell whether a man
is wise by his questions."

Naguib Mahfouz

DEFINITIVE POWER

"The power to define the situation is the ultimate power."
Jerry Rubin, activist and author (1938-1994)

As a political activist, it is likely Mr. Rubin meant that power derives from being able to define situations for others, thereby influencing their actions and reactions. And that is a great power indeed. This is the power of the Spin Doctor!

However, I believe a more practical meaning arises when I take this as the power to define the situation for myself. After all, the situation is only the situation. It is what it is. But the big questions are: What will the situation become? What do I do next?

My actions do not derive from the situation itself, my actions derive from my beliefs about what the situation demands. And as we all know, this varies a lot from person to person. Are my beliefs about this situation derived from my own worldview or were they shaped by others? Is my choice internal or external? Is it rigid or flexible? Am I acting or reacting?

In other words: Who's defining the meaning of the situation? Who's in control of my perceptions? Whoever this is, they control my direction.

Some people think it's impossible to shift your perceptions. If that were true, no one could intentionally change or redefine themselves. Don't believe everything you think!

I would add one thing to Mr. Rubin's quote: The power to define the situation is the ultimate power to facilitate my own growth.

And that's a power well within anyone's reach.

This quote reminds me of a 2000 year old saying:

"We are disturbed not by events, but by the views which we take of them." Epictetus, Greek philosopher, c.80AD

Today, while trying to verify that quote I kept finding this:

"It's not the events of our lives that shape us, but our beliefs as to what those events mean." Tony Robbins

Apparently two millennia ago people thought the author of this quote was Epictetus, but nowadays it's Tony Robbins. That's an interesting situation. What should I make of it?

It could be "everything old is new again." Or maybe "some things never change."

How about "there's nothing new under the sun" or even "talent borrows, genius steals!"

I guess it depends on which way I choose to perceive it.

THANK YOU

I am a therapist. It took a lot of time and effort to make this true. I graduated. I'm seeing clients. Bring on the rights and privileges thereto appertaining! I'm finding the things I get from being a therapist are the same things that brought me to it: Gifts and Miracles.

I've enjoyed the gift of fabulous teachers (which makes me a gifted student). I feel the best teachers do more than teach. The best teachers are also students. They engender skillful application and garnish it with an earnest quest for knowledge, thus enticing me to join. Be it professors, administrators, colleagues or supervisors, I've been blessed with the best from the best. I'm honored to say it's actually my job to pay this forward. And I'm proud to say, thanks to their generous tutelage, I'm increasingly capable of doing just that.

My father gave me the gift of humor. My mother the gift of intense focus and commitment. I have struggled to balance the two and now I bring this balance into the room.

My clients model strength, vulnerability, courage, trust and on occasion, miracles. They expose me and challenge me to be more aware, less defensive and more authentic. They push me to be better as I strive to better serve them. They give so bounteously I almost feel guilty collecting a fee. Almost. The fee keeps me mindful to repay the gifts I'm receiving. I do this by offering clients a present in exchange for their gifts. I offer them the gift of presence.

Clients are a miraculous gift, but no one has taught me more about manifesting miracles than my dear wife, Sherri. Whereas I'm basically a Type A, she is more of a Type C: Courageous, Creative and Congruent. But these are just her gifts, let me tell you about the miracle: Years ago, the best medical advice left us no reasonable expectation of a first anniversary. Yet here she is, with me at the culmination of a journey she in large part facilitated. We faced a difficult choice: focus on living what life we had left or focus on the problem threatening it. We chose to live our life fully, and by focusing on life we created more of it. Every day is a gift. This is our miracle. And a new gift is created every time we share it.

Since high school I wanted to be a therapist but I kept hearing, "People only go into psychology to solve their own problems." Stigma kept me away. Ultimately I pursued it. Now, with benefit of hindsight I revisit the question: Do people become therapists to work on their own issues? You bet your Asperger's they do. I certainly did. And thank God! Becoming a therapist enabled me to make tremendous personal progress. Crucial progress. It did so by providing me one thing I desperately needed: Plausible Deniability. Becoming a therapist requires committing to a substantial course of personal therapy without having to admit there is a problem. I knew I had things to work on, I just wasn't ready to know I knew it. By deciding to walk this path I was empowered to take the steps I needed to become the person (and the therapist) I always believed I could be. Along the way a fabulous job materialized, seemingly out of nowhere, which smoothed my road considerably. Apparently the universe was ready to admit I had a problem even if I wasn't quite there yet, and in my moment of need the universe offered a hand. What a miracle. What modeling! What an amazing gift to receive.

I'm filled with gratitude and every day it grows (well, most days). And how could it not? My appointment book is a bouquet of intimate moments. My colleagues are a network of skilled empathizers. My cost of doing business is self-care and personal development. In the service of helping others I help myself. Where else could I find a situation where I get so much value for giving so much value? I learn. I grow. I love to inspire. I am a therapist.

I COULDN'T HAVE SAID IT BETTER

People frequently tell me "That's exactly what I mean," and "I couldn't say it as well as you did." I'm not sure that's accurate. The truth is: You are saying it. Loudly and clearly!

That's why I can hear it and feed it back to you.

It's not that you can't say it, it's that you can't hear it… which makes it hard to act on it. When I feed it back to you in a way that's precise, concise and definite… now you hear it! Now you can take it and run with it wherever it goes.

You have the clarity to activate.

That's what therapy is about. Everyone is qualified to run the human race successfully. I simply help the runners hear the starter's gun more clearly.

Passion ☯ Perspective

"Nothing is so firmly believed as
what is least known."

Michel de Montaigne

"If something's true, you don't have
to believe in it."

Lily Tomlin

"No amount of belief makes
something a fact."

James Randi

TRUTH & THE ULTIMATE LIE

"No man, for any considerable period, can wear one face to himself and another to the multitude, without finally getting bewildered as to which may be true." Nathaniel Hawthorne, writer (1804-1864)

I believe this to be a fundamental aspect of communication: Whenever I speak to another I also speak to myself. This is why sarcasm is the ultimate lie. Sarcasm is the act of saying the opposite of what you mean while adding enough inflection to make it conspicuous. If I'm constantly reversing my meaning, I may eventually confuse myself and ultimately lose touch entirely with who I am.

"If you do not tell the truth about yourself you cannot tell it about other people." Virginia Woolf, writer (1882-1941)

I launched the process of becoming a therapist with one clear intention: to be an excellent therapist. This process changed me in many ways, one of the most notable being a dramatic drop in my use of sarcasm. I think Virginia's quote is an excellent explanation of why.

Being a good therapist has a lot to do with the truth. And the great thing about the truth is… everybody's got one!

FLOW OF LIFE

"I cannot prevent the wind from blowing, but I can adjust my sails to make it work for me."   Code of the Order of Isshinryu

There is a flow to the universe which happens regardless of our actions. This flow goes by many names: Natural order, God, Cause & effect, Karma, Physics, Fate, etc.

But flow it does, leaving us only one choice: join it or resist it.

When I resist I get very busy. The world abounds with opportunities to spend my energy. This gives me the illusion I'm getting somewhere. Swimming up-river is a lot of work, but it's a very inefficient use of time & effort.

It's easy to work hard, but working smart tends to be more productive. Working hard in smart directions should be unstoppable. So... what should I work on?

How about getting in touch with this flow? If I work hard on recognizing the flow, I can learn to drift with it and get "there" faster. I'm freer when I release my destination and learn to focus on where I'm heading... particularly when my heading needs to change.

If my goal is to arrive in only one place, I can fill my life with lots of work and the constant feeling I'm not there yet.

On the other hand, if my goal is to explore and express my true fundamental desires, I'm always being where I'd most like to be and I'll still wind up somewhere. Surprisingly, this formula leads to many wonderful places and a more enjoyable journey as well.

OK, so how do I identify my true fundamental desires?

That, my friend, is an entirely other article.

FRINGE BENEFITS

As you may know, I love being a therapist. It's not just the money, what really attracts me is the benefits package. Specifically, I like the professional exchanges I experience in this community, and I mean "exchange" in the broadest sense including occasional upsets and eruptions. Things come up when people work together. Shifts happen! But they happen differently in our world. I can think of one example in particular which illustrates my point.

Over time I noticed a colleague seemed more distant, less connected than usual. So as not to be paranoid I chalked it up to a number of things, none of which were my responsibility. Finally she pulled me aside and explained how several of our recent exchanges left her feeling uncomfortable (and at times a bit attacked). Knowing this was never my intention I became a tad defensive and received this feedback with active skepticism. I also did some creative blame-storming to assuage my discomfort with this news.

In many work settings the story could end right there, or more likely lead to ongoing "bad blood" or some sort of passive-aggressive drama. Not here though, because this was someone whose perception I trusted and respected. I reexamined our history and my behavior. I began to see I *was* acting oddly toward her, and in ways reflecting feelings I ultimately identified as frustration and anger. But none of her behavior seemed to warrant these feelings in any reasonable way, and I hate being unreasonable. So I looked a little further back and then I remembered something interesting.

A while ago I ran into her shortly after what I felt was a particularly fabulous session. I shared my enthusiasm over doing a good job in the room and she immediately shot back, "You know it's the client that did all the work, right?" All the wind drained instantly from my sails. I know it's true, but there was something in the way I heard it that really stung. I was very hurt and I believe a little angry as well. To her credit, she contacted me the very next day to apologize for the disheartening response which was definitely not her intention. I really appreciated this and let it go, or so I thought.

But the truth is I wasn't just hurt or angry, I was triggered. This is why my feelings hung around and resurfaced later. It wasn't about her comment, it was about a narcissistic injury from childhood (my mother is a very accomplished narcissist). This is my plight as the only living therapist who sprang from a narcissistic parent. Upon realizing I'd been triggered and that latent anger was motivating my behavior, I contacted my colleague and set up a meeting. I apologized for my behavior and explained the anger I carried from our earlier encounter. Believing I'd forgiven her afterward, I hadn't revisited these feelings but there they were, showing up in some rather inappropriate ways. After I recalled the original event admitting my feelings of deflation and anger she said the most amazing thing. She told me that she too had been triggered by that first encounter. She shared with me how when I first walked up, all full of my success, it brought to mind her narcissistic father and triggered her own narcissistic injury. The symmetry was astounding. I walked up and triggered her dad and she blithely returned the favor by triggering my mom. Just like in the textbooks. We each reacted true to form, caught in a game of dueling narcissists (each with our own parental banjo). But thanks to courage, awareness and a mutual willingness/desire to go deeper and get to the truth we worked it all through. This is what I call a successful professional exchange, one in which we both benefit.

In other careers my exchanges have led to improved products and techniques. I get that here too, but now I also become a more aware person in the process. I inherit this benefit simply by maintaining my place in the therapeutic community. In a client we might see this as secondary gain, but I assure you my gain is primary.

THE LATEST ADDICTION

There is a lot of press lately on Social Media addiction and the evil this engenders.

This is typical of news coverage today. Blame the symptom instead of the cause. They cite the number of addicts but never the number of people using the "addictive substance" who are not addicted (which does not support their claim).

I believe behavioral addiction is primarily an issue in the individual, the specific activity chosen to express the addiction is secondary. It makes a better story to blame new social trends but isn't it interesting that addiction has always existed while many addictive outlets are relatively new?

It's process over content once again. IMHO, we need to treat the underlying mechanism in operation and not focus so much on the particular expression if we want to make real progress with recovery issues.

I'm not sure the media is helping us in that regard. But recovery counselors and treatment specialists need to remember that's not the media's job... it's ours!

Passion ☯ Perspective

Past experience contributes to us
but needn't define us. Never let the
weight of the past become great
enough to limit growth.

Whenever I 'should' myself,
it's not my voice I'm hearing.

Maturity is not the negation
of childhood, but rather the
integration of it.

HOUSE BREAKING MY PET PEEVES

"I don't like that man. I must get to know him better."
                Abraham Lincoln, 16th U.S. President

Lincoln makes a cogent point in favor of self-knowledge. When my first reaction to someone is revulsion, it's more likely a statement about me than about them. After all, I hardly know them. So what am I bringing to the table here?

Quick intense judgments are frequently an indicator of deeper reactions. Be they Buttons, Triggers or Pet Peeves, they show me how some innocuous thing going on right here and now is activating a long standing irritant I'm carrying deep inside me…

Which is fantastic! Here's a golden opportunity to reveal a facet of myself of which I'm obviously unaware. Don't miss this opportunity! This is my take on President Lincoln's wisdom.

Or to put it another way, one of the surest paths to personal growth is this: When you spot a pet peeve, domesticate it!

TWO KINDS OF COLUMNS

I love New Years! A time of rebirth and renewal. I grab all my holiday gift cards and head to PsyMart for one of my favorite rituals: figuring out what I got this year. I decide to skip the cart for now and begin meandering up and down the aisles, drinking it all in. I'm here for the full experience! It's fun to check out the latest techniques, seeing what's hot and what's not. And the sales! I like to think of myself as a Master of PhD's (Post-holiday Discounts). I hope I'm in time to catch the cream of the crap. As I stroll along it occurs to me I'm not just looking at the shelves... I'm also checking out the other shoppers.

I glance in other people's carts as I pass, taking note of their selections and even eavesdropping on conversations now and then. I'm very curious about my fellow PsyMart shoppers. Suddenly a thought strikes me, piercing my holiday reverie like a bolt of lightning: There are two kinds of people in the world: People who divide the world into two kinds of people and people who don't. I see browsers and buyers. Cart fillers and hand carriers. Splitters and groupers? Hmmm, I guess it's pretty clear which path I chose at that particular fork in the road.

After years in the software industry I created "The 80/20 Theory of Programmers," a formulation for understanding software people which helps me address their needs more reliably. I muse for a moment on how programmers tend to view therapists. Then (since I sit on both sides of that fence) I drift to how therapists tend to view programmers. (a topic to which I'll return in a future column, but for now I must hasten back to PsyMart and my previous thread, because...)

Just then lightning strikes twice as a second (more relevant) thought comes to me: There are two kinds of therapists in the world, and there are many kinds of two kinds of therapists. There are dissectors and gestaltists, introverts and extroverts, confronters and comforters, processors and promoters. There are pathology based and strength based, single theory and eclectic (now integrative). There are therapists who want to help people and therapists who want to help themselves (and some that just can't help themselves). Indeed, therapists are fruitful fodder for playing "two kinds of people."

But "two kinds of people" is really just black and white thinking. Most truths (and people) lay somewhere in-between the extremes. Defining the poles simply delineates the scales by which we measure ourselves and each other. Sometimes I wonder if I come out more moderate on my scales than most others I assess. Possibly, but I shall examine my scales another time, for as we all know it is never appropriate to check your scales immediately after the holidays!

As therapists we are also familiar with the concept of shifting from content to process. So rather than examining the scales I return to the process of creating them. As I notice myself dividing people into types I recognize an important population to consider: clients. Do I split my clients into groups? "Two kinds of clients" can go many ways. Stimulating/Rote. Self-referred/mandated. Connected/Counter transferred. Contentious/Compliant. Insured/Self-pay. I'm concerned this game can take me away from my clients by reducing my presence. My clients and I will be better served if I scale back my "two kinds of people" time. Suffice it to say there are many kinds of two kinds of people, and of the two kinds of people I prefer the too kind people.

Now I'm traversing the aisles of PsyMart with a feeling of resolution. "Two kinds of people" is a game which yields valuable insights, they're just more about me than the people I set out to assess. Shopping at PsyMart is always satisfying. Amidst the vast, ever changing inventory there is one thing I can always count on finding: inspiration. I love being a therapist and if I ever decide to marry my job, we'll definitely register at PsyMart.

GROWTH IS NOT FOR EVERYONE

Growth is a process of increasing vulnerability. It's not for the defensive! As you open up you are certainly exposed to more pain, but don't let this limit your focus. You are also exposed to more love, compassion, wisdom, possibilities and joy! It's a fair tradeoff for the bold adventurer.

Growth is not for everyone, but it is always available to you.

NEW TECH, OLD FEAR

"The young people of today think of nothing but themselves. They have no reverence for parents or old age. They talk as if they knew everything, and what passes for wisdom with us is foolishness with them. As for the girls, they are forward, immodest and unladylike in speech, behavior and dress. When I look at the younger generation, I despair of the future of civilization."–Ancient Greece, 4th Century BC (personal attribution unclear)

People have always been saying the next generation will be the last. These crazy kids reject our values and engage in unwise activities which will inevitably unravel the very fabric of our society and leave us in ruin. This has been going on for over 2,000 years!

What's missing is the fact that each one of these younger generations actually becomes the older generation criticizing their younger generation. What's up with that?

The habits, fashions and technology of the younger generation are always topics for the older generation, inspiring reactions ranging from bewilderment to panic.

Today they say internet use and texting are destroying our ability to function socially. They said the same thing about the telephone over 100 years ago. New technology usually leads to a new equilibrium. When people say society will be destroyed, I wonder if they mean society will change. It could be the end of society *as we've known it*.

Perhaps the fundamental issue is the perception of a younger generation by an older one. Maybe the truth is we simply become more suspicious of change as we age.

New technologies come and go, but the fears they incite are perennial.

Passion ☯ Perspective

"An expectation is a down payment
on a resentment."

AA Wisdom

"Experience is what we get when
we don't get what we want."

Unknown

"Never forget there's a difference
between good sounding reasons and
good sound reasoning."

Unknown

FERTILE GROUND FOR THERAPY

The most fertile ground for therapy is the place where comfort and challenge blend harmoniously.

Comfort is an essential component of therapy. Without security and trust there is no safe place to open up and explore. But comfort alone invites stagnation. If I'm perfectly happy and cozy right where I am, why would I move?

Challenge is also essential to therapy. Without impetus and goals there will be no progress. But challenge alone invites resistance. I can only be pushed so far before I push back.

Comfort and Challenge. Both are needed. Neither is enough.

Good therapy finds a balance where each invites the other. That place where there's enough comfort to accept challenge and enough challenge to launch from comfort, thus creating the best opportunity for personal growth.

The optimal setting for therapy is where comfort and challenge achieve symbiosis.

DEAR ASPIRING PSYCHOTHERAPIST,

On a surface level you face a seemingly endless parade of pitfalls and annoyances that nip at your heels and invite you into resistance and discomfort. Do not RSVP!

Know that on a deeper level you are undertaking a heroic journey to become someone who authentically devotes their life to improving the world by soothing distress while increasing joy, acceptance and hope. You are not your paperwork, reading list and schedule. You are a healer in heart and spirit, soon to be validated in credential. You are walking a noble path. This is who you are and you prove it every day you go to work!

Your courage and commitment inspire me, may it do the same for you.

Sincerely,
HSW

YOURS, MINE AND HOURS

I remember having only a few hundred hours toward my 3000 and thinking "How will I ever get through this?" Now I have only a few hundred hours *remaining* and I think "How will I ever get through this?" I'm so anxious to be there already. I can get so focused on where I'm not it becomes hard to be where I am. I suffer from periodic absence of presence. Fortunately something always cycles me back.

Part of my job these days is training others to do the things I originally needed training to do. I face my fledgling therapist self at every step. I watch them struggle with the transition. They look to me for guidance and reassurance. Those were my eyes not so long ago. How much mirroring can one person stand? It pleases me that I've gained the confidence and experience to answer their questions, which I do most days at the center. Then I venture out into the land of private practice where I look to my supervisor, so established and accomplished. Once again I'm the one seeking all the answers. The cycle continues.

From my last career, to graduate school, to practicum and now toward licensure and practice. Transitioning out of a place I've grown comfortable, facing the loss while being excited about moving forward. Building comfort in a new circumstance while the next transition lurks on the horizon. I feel like a perpetual hatchling, just as my nest gets nice and cozy it's time to find a new one. During my practicum this center was my nest. I was nurtured and I grew and I deeply value this existence. Now that I'm comfy and established it's time to leave… and so it goes.

Cycles are omnipresent in every aspect of our work. There's the cycle that occurs with every client. A constant stream of new beginnings, the work goes how it goes and then we move on. In a single day I have many cycles in my journey from session to session; joining, processing and releasing in every meeting. Some of the work is simply keeping them straight. Being completely present on my client's path while in session and then stepping wholly off that path at the end. Clearing myself from one trail before joining the next client on another, or do the best I can.

There is another type of cycling I experience on a regular basis as I move forward in my journey: The cycling of my own self-image as a therapist. At first I was very closed down out of blind fear. After all, I don't want to ruin anybody's life. Then I started to gain confidence and began to let myself out a bit. As I did I found I didn't ruin anyone but I do have some rough edges and occasional triggers. When I catch myself triggered I reel myself in a bit and take my Counter Transference to therapy. After working it through and making some progress with these issues my confidence begins to increase. I expand myself as therapist once again and feel pretty good about it. Soon the next layer emerges and I get triggered anew. This is the most important cycle for me because this cycle enables C/T to become a tool for me rather than an impediment. My therapist has always said, "C/T is the greatest gift," but it's taken me years to unwrap it. There was nothing I studied more and understood less in my entire academic career. C/T is simply something that you have to experience to comprehend. Now I live it, note it, fear it, share it, work on it and ultimately come to respect and trust it. Then I'm ready for the next round.

The more things change the more they stay the same. This leg of my therapeutic journey is both exciting and terrifying. Once I get my license I naturally assume all my dreams will come true, but for now I have the luxury of knowing it's almost over…and then it will finally begin.

UPC: UNINTENDED PARENTAL CONSEQUENCES

In situations where parents are at odds or separated, it's not uncommon for one parent to criticize or diminish the other in the eyes of the child. It may be overt or covert… intentional or incidental… but it happens.

When it does, the criticizing parent may feel they are simply telling the truth (and in the process establishing they are the better parent). They may even feel they're helping the child feel safer by assuring them there is at least one caring/loving/responsible parent.

That is not what's actually happening.

Here is what's actually happening:

Every child knows they are the product of both parents. When one parent teaches the child there is something wrong with the other parent, the lesson the child learns is not "thank goodness I have at least one good parent." The lesson the child learns is "uh oh, if there's something wrong with one of my parents there is something wrong with me."

This is not a helpful lesson for any child.

Co-parenting is about support. Not just for the child, but for each other as well. That's a good lesson for anyone!

EXTRAORDINARILY AVERAGE

The average person is average. This is true for all walks of life and every field of endeavor.

If we subscribe to the theory that everyone is unique or special in some way, then every person has the potential to be extraordinary. Particularly the average person.

I believe the path to extraordinary runs right through the expression of the authentic self. A leap of awareness and honesty in being is all that's required. I have only to discover (or remember) more about myself.

The average person is not in touch with their extraordinary nature, but they could be.

Passion ☯ Perspective

"Should you shield the canyons from
the windstorms you would never see
the true beauty of their carvings."

Elisabeth Kubler-Ross

"Man is most nearly himself when
he achieves the seriousness of
a child at play."

Heraclitus

THE SPECIFICITY PARADOX

What is your client population? Who do you want to see? Who will you help?

These can be vexing questions for psychotherapists in general, particularly so for interns and trainees. These questions raise many emotions for us, chief among them is fear.

Here is a sample internal dialogue:

"If I'm too specific I may lose a lot of potential clients."

"Oh? Who are your potential clients?"

"Well, there's mood issues, anxiety, trauma, relationships, grief. Oh yeah, and eating disorders, OCD, social issues, work pressures and life transitions. Pretty much everyone."

"So you want to see everyone?"

"Of course not. But I don't want someone to read my ad and think I can't help them."

Aha! Fear of rejection. Which in this case is a mask for a fear of inability to launch my career. A career in which I've invested more years, $$$$'s and intimate personal resources than most professions come close to demanding. After this kind of commitment, I don't want anything to limit my ability to succeed!

So when I answer the question, "Who are my clients?" my main goal is avoiding rejection.

That makes sense psychologically, but it's a very poor strategy. Here's 2 reasons why:

1) In order to avoid rejection you are going to make your ad so generalized and so amorphous that no one will identify with it. Therefore, no one will see their issue in your description. Therefore no one will have any reason to think you can help them.

2) You can't see everyone! There isn't enough time in the week.

I'm afraid if I'm too specific about my primary client I'll miss too many potential clients. But to get clients I have to be specific enough to be chosen.

This is The Specificity Paradox!

Do you want clients? Then take this to heart:

Getting clients is not about avoiding rejection, it's about getting selected!!!

Getting clients is about reaching the 100 people in the area who need your help. It's not about keeping 1,000,000 people in the area from rejecting you.

You only need some clients. So when you answer these big questions, be as specific as possible. The people looking for you need to know you are the one they seek!

You can't see a million clients. But if you design your marketing to appeal to all of them you can easily wind up with none.

LIGHTS, CAMERA, INSIGHT!

Why did you become a therapist? As I write this I am crossing the 3,000 hour barrier and compiling my BBS application for MFT exam eligibility. I've been so busy getting these hours I frequently lose sight of why I'm doing it. Here's a few scenes from my "Why I became a therapist" montage...

Friends ask me what to do and I tell them. Complete strangers share intimate details because I'm "a person you can open up to." People at parties say, "that's what my therapist told me." It creeps into my work life. On movie sets I bolster actors through fragile moments to get better takes. As Engineering Manager I help programmers with their personal problems instead of sending them to classes or seminars, and they become more productive. It reaches the point where I'm being a therapist in every possible way except actually being a therapist. Finally I decide to take the plunge and enroll at JFK University. [We see HOWARD entering the JOHN F. KENNEDY UNIVERSITY building. As the door closes we SLOWLY DISSOLVE to: HOWARD sitting at a KEYBOARD wearing a CAP & GOWN]

"Yes, that was me 3,000 clinical hours ago. Back then I really thought I was being a therapist. Now I am a real therapist and I realize how back then I wasn't really being a therapist at all. But now that I'm an actual therapist, what becomes of the non-therapeutic me many of us thought was a therapist?"

That's the big question. Do I simply throw it out? The sum total of my acquired knowledge and techniques is what clients pay for. My old pseudo-therapist was indiscriminant and frequently clinically inappropriate. And there it is, boundaries and barriers rise again. Take that to the room. Keep this in the room. Get that out of the room. Propriety and discretion. Ethics and mindfulness should make it simple to sort out, yet every time I step into the room I inevitably bring all of it with me and sometimes that clouds the issue. Life experience, that's the magical stuff of which empathy, understanding and rapport are made… until it invites Counter-Transference. C/T is a gift but not if I get triggered. And what of my pet peeves? Those little buttons which can turn me from a therapist into a thera-pissed. I recycle many a fee through my own therapist in order to transform them into domesticated pet peeves, then I set them free. This whole package comes with me (either intentionally or subliminally) wherever I go, particularly when I enter the room. Some of it useful, some not so much. One amazing thing about this package is how it can change from day to day, sometimes in very dramatic ways, just as it did for me recently…

Let me share what happened with a very important piece of *my* life experience: my wife, Sherri. A while ago I wrote about how well she's been doing since her terminal diagnosis in 2008, and about three days after that was published she suffered a massive relapse. Given the 1% survival rate for late stage esophageal cancer, this was very scary to say the least. She underwent chemo and radiation, then we had to wait. Finally we were cleared for a PET scan to gauge the progress. When the results arrived, we saw the scan was totally clear. No detectable traces of cancer at all. Sherri is in remission! It's astounding, we have literally experienced a miracle! We now live in a world of infinite possibility and the genuine knowledge that everything is going to be fine and will work out as it should… which is great for Sherri and me.

But I think it's great for my clients as well. Bringing this kind of energy into the room seems a powerful intervention. My challenge is to preserve it in affirmative empathy for my clients. To be lovingly present in the knowledge that we're doing the best we can in the moment and are exactly where we should be, but also knowing this in no way limits us from heading directly and exactly where we need to go.

I think I'm clear about why I became a therapist, but I find my view of what therapy is keeps evolving and changing. In this moment I see therapy as a race to stay on track and not get tethered conceptually. Navigating mazes of emotions and ideas, the challenge is remaining undistracted by content, by C/T or by defenses (theirs or mine). To stay clean and clear through all this toward the actual point of healing. That's the journey. Along the way you bring everything you have and ideally that toolkit is constantly growing, often in the most beautiful ways.

IS THERAPY CONFRONTATIONAL?

Depending on the therapist, their style and the particular issue involved, a client's experience in therapy may or may not feel confrontational.

Being a therapist, however, is very much about confrontation.

If you want to be an effective therapist you must confront your fears and you must confront yourself, both your relational and your actual self. You must confront your past, your limits and your defenses. You must emerge as who you genuinely are before you can credibly ask someone else to do the same.

I say that you must do these things, but the truth is you don't have to do any of these things at all. You don't have to be an effective therapist either.

Passion ☯ Perspective

Some people erase past relationships,
creating a fresh clean slate for the
next one… then they proceed
to draw the exact same picture.

As we alter patterns we inspire
fresh directions.

Sometimes when people ask
your opinion, all they really want is
your blessing.

MIND OVER SPLATTER

I have a very cute dog with a lovely, upbeat disposition (which is quite charming). A little less so when he needs to be walked. Less still when it's raining. And on a day like today when I have to arrive on time to an all-day training, his lackadaisical sense of timing on walks can be downright irritating. It's like he has no respect for my schedule. And after all I've done for him!

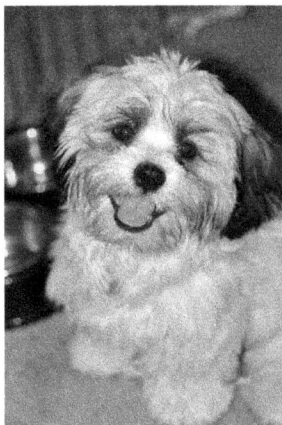

So we're trudging along through the pitter patter of the raindrops and the splitter splatter of the mud-puddles and I'm really into being annoyed. At this moment, the dog that I love is a nuisance and an impediment.

Fortunately, this is day 2 of a seminar on experiential techniques which are all about being aware in the moment and opening new possibilities. So instead of just being annoyed I start to pay attention to the how and why of my annoyance and I revisit my situation.

Here I am, walking early in the morning with no one else around (courtesy of the rain). A peaceful placid stroll, listening to some of my favorite music. Here's Jack, the wonder-puppy, bobbing along in his typically jubilant gait. He's pretty happy at the moment, begging the question: How am I not? I look at Jack again, only this time I decide to let go of the nuisance lens and instead see him as I usually do: my floppy goofball compatriot. Suddenly all my irritation dissolves. My heart swells with joy and I am incredibly happy.

And all I did was switch my focus from one aspect of the current moment to another.

I think seminars and trainings can be very useful, but it's amazing what you can learn from your puppy.

ROLL CONFUSION

I undertook this column knowing full well my primary goal as a pre-licensee (much like a therapist) is to obsolete myself. And now my role as pre-licensee is drawing to a close. This got me thinking about roles and the role I want to talk about today is payroll! Something happened recently in private practice. My supervisor and I discovered something very significant. Something every intern/supervisor pair in private practice needs to understand.

First a brief review: When a supervisor brings an intern into private practice, the intern must be an employee and there must be an agreement as to how the intern will be paid. All fees go directly to the supervisor (by law) and the supervisor divvy's up the proceeds as outlined in their agreement. Many supervisors like having interns but they don't like having employees (because of paperwork and taxes), so they hire a payroll service to handle that part and everyone is happy. Such is the case with my supervisor and me.

Here's what happened next: When I got my first pay stub from the payroll service, I noticed my gross pay was reduced. I asked my supervisor about this and she said this is how they've always done it. We wrote to the payroll service and they explained the reduction. They take the "Employer Payroll Tax" out first and then do the regular payroll processing on the remainder. I asked them, "Shouldn't the Employer pay the Employer Payroll Tax?" They said most of their clients are MFTs or LCSWs and 90% of them handle it exactly this way and *they recommend we do it too*.

So my supervisor and I decided to take some consultation and several things emerged. First, Employers are indeed responsible for Employer Payroll Taxes (it's *illegal* to have the employee pay them). Second, the topic of Employer Payroll Taxes rarely comes up when making a supervisor/intern fee split agreement. Third, most MFT's and interns are not very financially sophisticated, particularly when it comes to tax laws or employment stuff, which is why... fourth, most supervisors hire payroll services which may set up situations just like this. I think we're all clear that MFTs are not doctors, lawyers and especially not tax accountants. Seriously, how many of us need help just counting our BBS hours? But who *should* know better about something like this?

I'm not into blaming here, not until I do more research, but the fact remains this payroll service asked my supervisor for only one number: the employee's (my) share of the fees. Then they took the Employer Payroll Taxes out of that portion. They were the ones responsible for allocating these payments. In my opinion, *they* should know better than to take the Employer Payroll Taxes from the Employee's share. Every supervisor and intern should know this too. According to CAMFT, this is illegal and creates a potential liability for the supervisor. I wonder if this is why many qualified MFT's elect not to host interns in private practice?

You can make an open agreement to deal with the tax however you like, but you can't split the gross and then take the Employer Payroll Tax out of the employee's share.

I believe supervisors and interns are unaware of these rules. I'm proud to say my supervisor had the integrity to pursue this directly and see it through to an ethical and appropriate conclusion. Thank you, Maria. I never doubted it but I so appreciate it.

HERE'S THE PROBLEM WITH...

There is a certain kind of person with which we're all familiar. They always know what's wrong with something. Be it a product, circumstance or popular issue, they know why it's a mess and they know it won't get fixed.

It could be fixed (they'll tell you precisely how), but they know it won't be fixed because the powers that be can't see it as clearly as this person does.

When smart people focus on problems and blockages, they tend to see what doesn't work. Frequently these people wind up doing nothing. Of course that's not how they see it. In their view, they are saving effort and energy by never running down blind alleys. They feel pride in their tremendous efficiency.

I believe it's more likely they are just shortchanging their life's potential. These people are stuck. So, what should you do about it? Avoid them?

No. Learn from them.

Take advantage of a wonderful opportunity. Think of how you react to things. Find times when you agree with their hopelessness about a situation and pay attention. Let them help you see where you may be stuck...

Then free yourself.

Passion ☯ Perspective

"Too often we underestimate the
power of a touch, a smile, a kind word,
a listening ear, an honest compliment,
or the smallest act of caring,
all of which have the potential
to turn a life around."

Leo Buscaglia,

WHERE TRUTH LIES

"Art is not truth. Art is a lie that makes us realize truth."

Pablo Picasso

This is a very powerful concept and one of my favorite quotes. Its interest lies in the questions it raises.

If a lie reveals truth, is it really a lie? And how then do we judge the liar? Is it ethical to lie when the goal is to lead rather than mislead? Is it OK ever? Never? Only when it works?

Does this mean artists are liars? Are they people who invite truth without ever expressing it?

One of the great things about truth is that everybody's got one! When practicing artistry, which truth is relevant?

In the therapy world, Strategic Family Therapists are devoted to Picasso's perspective. They use a technique called paradoxical interventions. The therapist makes you promise to obey without question, then assigns an absurd sounding task which seems more likely to worsen the issue than cure it. In practice, if the client follows through, this frequently breaks down resistance and precipitates healthier outcomes. When done skillfully (perhaps artfully) this is a very effective technique.

Instead of dealing with you openly they mislead you to a solution. It sounds odd, but it's done thoughtfully and very carefully. Nonetheless, it does beg the question: Is it appropriate for a therapist to lie to you if it helps you find the truth?

What if it helps you find and comprehend your truth? Isn't this the job of a therapist? I believe it truly is.

Fortunately, paradoxical interventions are only one of many ways to get there.

And that's no lie.

GIVING THANKS FOR GRATITUDE

New beginnings happen all the time. I'm having several right now. I'm launching so many new directions I was going to write about transitions, but I was blocked. I was stuck in my head and I couldn't make it work. Then I remembered it's Thanksgiving, time to honor a lesson for which I am most thankful: speak authentically from your heart. Right now, my heart is full of gratitude. It occurs to me gratitude is a great way to begin anything. So let's begin with a big one:

I didn't write a column last issue because we had issues. After four years of torturous treatments and roller coaster relapses, Sherri (my wife) had major surgery attempting to cure her cancer. After months of slow painful progress, all indications now point to success and Sherri may well be cancer free. A 50-to-1 shot! I cannot begin to describe how incredibly grateful I am for this blessing on so many levels.

I am thankful for the wisdom of my teachers, mentors, supervisors and colleagues. When I speak in the room I frequently hear their voices in my head, guiding me (just to be clear, those voices are definitely *inside* my head… and they're gently guiding, *not* critiquing or commanding). I sincerely hope to honor them by channeling this wisdom in the service of my clients.

I'm grateful for the internal work I've done on this journey. People say this path changes you. They are so right! I truly believe the process of striving to be a competent therapist has made me a healthier person. And on the topic of being a healthier person…

I have an amazing therapist. For years she has mirrored, modeled, managed, contained and supported me. She showed me how a therapeutic relationship can grow and evolve and flourish. She helped me realize great gifts and she inspires me to inspire others.

I am eternally grateful for her counsel and caring. I owe so much to her. I am, however, current in my fees.

And I am grateful for clients. They invite us to be brilliant for them and sometimes we rise to the occasion and create magical moments of healing… here is one that comes to mind for me: I was seeing an elementary school boy who had recently lost his mother to cancer. I asked him if he felt his mother inside him and he said no, there was just a big empty space. An idea struck me and I asked him to get some Play-Doh and a sand tray figure to represent his mom (he chose Olive Oyl, Popeye's girlfriend). I had him press Olive face-down into the Play-Doh and I asked him: "Is this how you and your mom used to be together?" and he shook his head yes. Then I pulled out the Olive figure and showed him the Play-Doh, indicating the empty space. "Is this how you feel now?" He said yes. Then I held it up so he could look directly into the impression in the Play-Doh. "Can you see Olive Oyl's face and clothes in the Play-Doh?" and he said yes. Then I said, "You know that empty space inside you? I'll bet your mom is in there just like Olive Oyl is in here." I don't know where that came from but it was one of those remarkable moments in the room. I can't remember another job where moments like this could happen any day.

After literally thousands of hours in the room I still find this work intensely compelling. The intimacy, the growth and the potential for discovery are amazing aspects of my workplace.

I'm also grateful you are reading this. After all, writing exclusively for myself is just journaling, and that only goes so far.

Last but not least, I'm grateful for PsyMart, the therapist's ultimate shopping experience. Next issue is New Year's, which is always PsyMart shopping time. I can hardly wait to see what's on sale!

PAINFUL LESSONS

"To hurry pain is to leave a classroom still in session. To prolong pain is to remain seated in a vacated classroom and miss the next lesson." Yahia Lababidi

How long should grieving last? When will I feel better?

These are tough questions because the pain is very real. Working through and recovering from loss is a very important process. On the other hand, relieving symptoms quickly and moving on has a lot of value too. When I'm in emotional pain I want to know: How long do I have to go through this? Are we there yet?

Sometimes the pain seems too much to bear. I may need a break before facing difficult times. A little instant relief has tremendous appeal. This is why substance use remains such a time honored tradition in the human condition... it works! Be it booze, drugs, food, work or gambling. It doesn't matter what vehicle I choose. What matters is understanding this: When I anesthetize difficult feelings I don't heal them, I merely put them on hold.

So, if my break lasts for days or weeks, this may be very helpful in arresting the pain. But if my break lasts for years and my use turns to abuse, then the only thing I'm arresting is my own development.

Think of it like this: Moving through a difficult loss or adjustment is more than a healing process, it is also a growth process. Healing is about feeling better but growth is about being better. Ultimately we seek both, as completely as possible.

How fast can I heal? It depends on my health, outlook and the quality of my support system.

How fast can I grow? It depends on my personality and life timing.

So how do I measure my grief process progress? Unfortunately it's very hard to say, but one thing is clear: To move forward I must earnestly engage the growth process, which means engaging my feelings (not avoiding them) and facing the fundamental truth of grieving:

The only way out… is through.

Passion ☯ Perspective

"Placing blame in marriage is like saying, 'Your side of the boat is sinking.'"

Hank Smith

"Contempt is the weapon of the weak and a defense against one's own despised and unwanted feelings."

Alice Miller

CHOOSING CHANGE

Change. Some say it's the only constant.

Change is what we want when we don't want to be where we are. Change is what therapy is all about. No one hires a therapist to keep things as they are.

Choices are at the root of all change. Whether they are my choices or not. Whether they are conscious choices or unconscious. Every choice closes some doors and opens others. This changes my landscape of possibilities. It redefines my available choices.

That's change!

It's hard to predict all the consequences of our choices, to know what change we are creating. It may be easier to simply ask if the choice reflects my own desires and needs. Am I making this choice from my internal compass or to gain the approval of others? Are the two in conflict? Do I even know the difference?

One thing's for sure: Change will happen.

Each choice invites change and each change poses new choices, this is the circle of life.

Learning to make choices which honor my integrity, this is the nature of growth.

A PSY OF RELIEF...

Nothing says Happy New Year like taking my harvest of gift cards down to PsyMart (Costco for therapists). Upon arrival, the parking lot tells me I'm not alone in my post-holiday reverie. I take the first available space… 3 miles from the entrance. I grab a stray cart (sensing they may be scarce) and start rattling along. It occurs to me people come to therapists to lose baggage but therapists come to PsyMart to gain baggage. That's why the carts are so big!

But how shall I fill mine? My best gift this holiday (after a healthy wife) was from the BBS! As a newly licensed therapist I'm open to many possibilities. There is, however, one must-have item today: a shiny new mirror for my new office. Once inside the store I approach the nearest PsyMart Customer Experience Facilitator for some help…

"Hello sir, what brings you to PsyMart today?"

"Can you direct me to the mirrors?"

"Certainly, you'll find them at the end of your true path."

"Can you direct me to my true path?"

"You're on it."

Hmmm. A glance at her nametag confirms my suspicions: "Hello, I'm Debbie, PsyMart Non-Directive Associate." I courteously externalize myself from the conversation and venture out into acres of sprawling merchandise.

After a while I find myself in the Boundary Friendly gift section. An "Answers to Common Client Questions" calendar catches my eye. I pick up the display model and start flipping pages…

January 5, What is therapy? *Therapy is a journey you take by yourself….with me.*

February 14, What's a healthy couple supposed to be like? *In a healthy couple each partner feels they're getting the best of the bargain.*

March 17, How come you know all about me and I don't know anything about you? *You know that I listen to you. You know I care about your safety and well-being. You know I work to understand you as best I can and I'm always there for you (at least within 24 hours). You may not be clear on a few details but it sounds like you know some very important things about me.*

April 1, What's normal? *A normal person is someone you just don't know very well.*

Ah yes, April Fools Day. But I can't spend all year on this calendar (at least not today), so I toss a fresh one in my cart and press on through the plethora. Where are those mirrors?

I pass through Experiential Interventions, Focused Intentions, Theoretical Inventions and Anxieties & Apprehensions (which naturally shares an aisle with Processing Tensions). Finally I reach my destination, the PsyMart Mirror department, where therapists come to reflect. It's hidden between Art Therapy Supplies and Cognitive Notions (amidst frames and reframes).

A mirror may not sound ideal for someone (like myself) who is still retaining a lot of holiday cheer, but PsyMart has remarkable mirrors. While gazing into one I notice I've lost some psychic weight. Upon reflection I realize how I used to take more of a tornado approach, busting up the status quo and forcing change where I felt it was needed. Perhaps I just needed an aftermath to feel some validation. Now I see how I've mellowed. Now I aspire to be the rolling breeze, the only evidence of my visit being new ships safely moored in previously unreachable ports. I feel much better as the "winds of change," it's a big step up from "blow hard." Yes, this is my mirror. And it's slimming, too! I pop it in the cart and head for checkout…

Which is chaos! Enormous lines. Overflowing carts everywhere. But one lighted sign beckons: "Express Check Out: Licensed 5 Years or Less." Incredible, my brand new license is already paying dividends. After years of intensely focused effort I have reached the culmination of my journey. Now that it's finished I am finally free to begin. Standing here on the threshold of my first year of licensure, I'm setting intentions to make it an excellent one. The first of many! Happy New Year!

CRANIAL CONSTRUCTION ZONE

Your brain is the last of the body's major organs to become complete. In fact, it does not finish developing until approximately age 25.

This becomes even more interesting when we consider how many significant life decisions we make before age 25. These decisions were made by a brain still under construction, which could explain a lot.

Some people think this means the brain is one of the slowest developing organs in the body, but I don't see it that way. I think the brain is just so incredibly awesome that it takes longer to finish the project.

And I'm thinking this with a brain that was finished quite a while ago.

Passion ☯ Perspective

"If liberty means anything at all,
it means the right to tell people
what they do not want to hear."

George Orwell

"You can be kind with the truth or
blunt with the facts."

Ruth Ann Auten, MFT

POTENTIAL REALIZATION

Everyone has potential. At any given moment each of us is realizing some percentage of that potential, and it's never 100%. Whether it's 16% or 92% we can always do better. Perfectionists are obsessed with this idea, but I don't recommend that.

I recommend considering how much of your own potential you are currently realizing. Not judging yourself about it, but simply paying attention. It's an interesting statement about how you're currently doing and who you currently are.

If it feels a little low these days, it's reasonable to consider bumping it up a bit. You might ask yourself: Why am I not taking more responsibility for utilizing my potential?

Frequently the answer comes down to either Ease or Fear.

Let's face it, cruising is easy. If I'm enjoying a leisurely pace and still doing OK, there may not be much motivation to change. It's about quality of life.

Fear, of course, is not so easy. We are each of us endowed with huge potential. But living up to that potential can be very intimidating. This thought may ease the burden:

I give a gift to the world when I realize my potential and share it. Yet the rewards I receive far exceed any I give. This isn't about quality of life, it's about quality of life-experience!

Perhaps Marianne says it best:

"Our deepest fear is not that we are inadequate. Our deepest fear is that we are powerful beyond measure. It is our light, not our darkness that most frightens us. We ask ourselves, 'Who am I to be brilliant, gorgeous, talented, fabulous?' Actually, who are you not to be? Your playing small does not serve the world. There is nothing enlightened about shrinking so that other people won't feel insecure around you. We are all meant to shine, as children do... And as we let our own light shine, we unconsciously give other people per-mission to do the same. As we are liberated from our own fear, our presence automatically liberates others."

Marianne Williamson, A Return to Love: Reflections on the Principles of "A Course in Miracles"

THE SIGNIFICANCE OF OUR OTHERS

What's on the agenda for today? Agendas! And in honor of Valentine's Day I'm thinking of one in particular: The Love Agenda.

February 14th is the one day of the year our agenda for love is clear. Flowers, candy, lovely cards and a romantic dinner. We know the routine (and judging by the prices, so do the vendors). But what about the other 364 days of the year? Who sets our love agenda then? And what are we trying to achieve?

Perhaps we just follow our hearts, as French philosopher Blaise Pascal suggested long ago: "The heart has its reasons which reason knows nothing of." What a lovely Valentine's sentiment. The brain doesn't know what that wacky heart is up to. This is the plot basis of most romantic comedies, our bastion of societal lore about love. There is a lot of "story" about love. Perhaps on Valentine's Day story goes hand-in-hand with agenda.

But I don't think Blaise was talking about love, I think he was talking about unconscious motivation. It seems to me we set many of our agendas beneath conscious awareness. This takes me to some interesting places. Won't you join me, please...

Here's a big question: How do we select partners? There are the obvious answers: love, compatibility, romance, sexuality, loneliness, money, convenience, etc. Lately I'm struck with another idea, PC. I believe we always make Perfect Choices in partners.

Next question: How do these relationships work out? Good enough to keep many of us in business. So much for perfection, eh? Well, consider this...

What are these perfect choices for? Not love. Not procreation. We make perfect choices for our growth. We choose partners who inspire us to move toward higher developmental ground. We pick partners who trigger us in just the right way (although it may not feel like it in the moment).

Next consider how we don't always know why we're making these perfect choices. The choices are usually made by our unconscious which is more familiar with our growth needs than we are. Is there a more powerful radar system than unconscious desire?

Finally, remember the difference between opportunity and action. Our perfect choices merely identify and select possibilities for growth. We knock on the door but when someone answers we still face the challenge of growth. This is a separate choice. We don't always go for it. It depends on our current agenda.

Perfect Choices can be a helpful perspective for framing couples work. Of course, the true test of a perspective is in the framing. Perfect Choices sees "Opposites Attract" as an example of two people choosing large growth challenges or taking a bold step toward balance. "The Honeymoon is Over" may reveal the moment we begin releasing fantasy/projection and start to face the actual growth challenge we've selected, or perhaps this is the first time we're triggered by a partner. "I keep winding up with the same kind of person," can indicate a client who is stuck at a crucial growth step.

Perfect Choices is an agenda. It is a love agenda (frequently an unconscious one) but Perfect Choices is also an agenda for growth. I find Perfect Choices to be a convenient and affirmative way to frame couple issues in the room. It can serve as a framework for helping clients bring mindful awareness to previously hidden motives and goals, and that's a major part of *my* agenda as a therapist.

"The heart has its reasons which reason knows nothing of." In the extreme, one might insist we are always better off when dealing overtly with genuine motivations. Only making clear conscious choices and bringing all unconscious shenanigans into the light. No impulse goes unacknowledged and no agenda is hidden! I'm not sure this is achievable. In fact, this is possibly the agenda of a cosmic control freak. For my own agenda, simply helping clients disarm their triggers and receive the gifts of growth they are seeking… this is a therapeutic challenge I can accept.

EMOTIONAL BAGGAGE BELLHOP

We are all bellhops in the Hotel of Life. The more baggage we carry, the fewer doors we can fit through.

The real burden of emotional baggage is the toll it takes on our possibilities. It's one of life's great distractions. When we think of distracted drivers we tend to think of the risks and dangers, but what about the great stops we miss? These are lost opportunities that could make our trip richer and more memorable.

Similarly in life, I can be so busy servicing my baggage that I miss valuable experiences or chances for personal development. I limit myself in more ways than I know. How can I count what I don't even notice?

I'm taking the trip either way, must I minimize its value?

At its root, emotional baggage is ironic. How can something so easy to carry be such a heavy burden?

Gratitude, curiosity, forgiveness and responsibility are useful tools for releasing the pieces of emotional baggage we carry.

As a bellhop in Hotel Life, I'm better off dumping bags whenever I can. The goal is being able to reach every room in the place so I won't miss any big tippers. And don't worry about making a mess, Hotel Life is blessed with an amazing housekeeping staff.

Passion ☯ Perspective

Justifying myself is not accepting myself.

Judging lets us deal with a problem without taking responsibility for changing it. Condemning myself excuses me from improving myself.

PAYING BEETHOVEN WHAT HE IS ODE

I saw a YouTube video of a spontaneous Beethoven's 9th Flash Mob at Banco Sabadell. It brings tears to my eyes each time I see it. It starts so simply and builds and builds as flash mobs do… but as this one progresses I see (and feel) joy and inspiration spreading and captivating the onlookers. I can see it in their faces and actions. No one just sits and listens. They are literally *moved*.

I believe this displays some fundamental components of healing: surprise, delight, spontaneity and the creation by a few people of a great beauty that reaches out and touches many others. When a critical mass of positivity is achieved, awesome healing power is generated.

This is one way to approach therapy, helping people reconstruct just such a core of positivity in at least one aspect of their life. As it takes hold, this joy spreads bit by bit to fill and revitalize their entire life.

It's a fun process building bridges to help people reconnect with concepts and ideals which may have fallen from view during a busy life. Some call this therapy. I like to think of it as Awareness Engineering.

By the way, the title of Beethoven's 9th Symphony:

"Ode to Joy."

STUDYING DOES NOT PRECLUDE LEARNING

As my wife shifts from patient to survivor (as all indicators portend), I find myself in transition from caretaker/advocate to grateful spouse. As I adjust to the challenges of private practice I'm redefining my community and my professional identity is in transition, being kneaded and tested. And then there's the transition to licensure. Interestingly, this transition highlights the role which never changes in my life: Student. And it was while studying for my first licensing exam that a funny thing happened... I learned something that can make me a better therapist.

Whenever I'd miss a practice question I'd scrutinize the answer rationale. Sometimes it was an oversight and sometimes it was a bad guess, but sometimes I was answering an entirely different question than the one asked. How did that happen?

After enough of these I realized that some questions just irritated me. In my search for a way to conquer the exam I developed a sense for how the exam questions *ought to be*. I was so smug about it that when a question didn't seem fair or reasonable to me (read: didn't match my expectation) I'd get angry at the question! Next I'd start telling myself a story about how the question *should have been* written and now I'm fighting the question rather than reading it. Then I'd select my answer based on my story about the question rather than the actual question itself. Ultimately I had to face the fact I was getting triggered by some of the exam questions.

"Seriously?!?!" I told my mirror, "You're triggered by the MFT exam? Isn't that unethical? Or illegal?" And the mirror said, "Ethical or legal, cite the difference!" I needed exam therapy...STAT!

I began to see how, when triggered, I tend to hold on to my story so tightly it clouds my vision. I knew I needed to let that go for the exam, but where else is this happening in my life?

Just as fighting questions keeps me from seeing, fighting reality keeps me from being. When I'm overly attached to outcomes, when I need my world to be a certain way… then I get very busy rejecting everything outside my rigid expectation. I get so busy rejecting that I miss the bounty available in each moment. Can I let my story go and relax into the present?

Baggage weighs us down and exhausts our playful spirit, the child who sees with open eyes. The child who remains unfettered by preconceptions, dictums and agendas. Releasing is such a large part of what I recommend to clients. "Whenever you release baggage you can fit through more doors." It wouldn't do me any harm either.

So the more I let go, the more I have? No, but perhaps the more I let go the more I am able to be. I'm free to acquire new things when my arms aren't full of old baggage.

We are always in transition. If nothing else we are always passing from moment to moment. Sometimes I think transitions are about picking a new destination and getting where you're going. But in order to get anywhere I must first let go of where I am. "Going" is an option, but "letting go" is mandatory. This means there may be a time when I've released where I was and haven't gotten where I'm going yet… that can be a very uncomfortable place. On the other hand, if I only set goals within my immediate grasp I may never get out of my neighborhood.

Transitions are a big deal to me because clients rarely come in seeking to stay where they are. Transition is what therapy is all about… and I am all about therapy.

When I consider my toolkit for dealing with transitions it occurs to me that maybe it isn't what I have but rather what I'm willing to release that's the greatest determinant of transitional success. Perhaps I should leave it at that, but I just have to say: Sometimes the biggest lessons come from the most surprising places. Who knew studying for licensing exams could be so educational?

PERFECTLY MISTAKEN

Mistakes are a topic worth repeating.

I relish mistakes. When learning something new I make as many mistakes as possible, as fast as possible.

My goal is not to avoid mistakes, my goal is to avoid repeating them!

Perfectionism is the opposite of making mistakes. It is a deadly trap. It shoehorns me into a repetitive rigidity which is very limiting... and somehow mistakes still happen! I might make fewer of them but I'm less likely to admit/tolerate them. This taxes my immune system and my spirit. It also makes me less likely to benefit from my mistakes.

Perfectionism is unhealthy. It is the opposite of growth. If you are never making mistakes, you simply aren't doing anything.

Show appreciation for your mistakes by fully realizing their value, especially when your mistake is perfectionism!

Passion ☯ Perspective

"When I seek approval outside myself,
I'm in trouble."

Marlene Decker, MFT

"Some people go to therapy, some
people go to graduate school."

Mary Crocker Cook, MFT

I'M PAST THAT NOW

Splitting vs Integrating is a very popular therapy topic.

Splitting is the problem: If there's a mistake or unappealing part of my past I simply eliminate it by saying "That wasn't me. I'm not like that." Then I go my merry way. Of course this part of me isn't gone. It will come back to haunt me when I get triggered, because there is no erasing a part of myself and there is nothing I have ever done that "wasn't me."

Integrating is the solution: The only way to become healthy is to make peace with parts of myself I don't like or thoughts/feelings/actions of which I'm ashamed. Integrating is the process of accepting the "unacceptable" parts of myself and being OK with the entirety of me.

Dr. Liz Zed, a great mentor gave me a great example of just how to do this. She says: "Everything I've ever done or been has contributed to who I am now. They were all steps on the journey to become me. I don't regret anything because I'm good with who I am and I look forward to what I'm becoming. Why would I regret anything that brought me here?"

AN ARTISTIC SCIENCE

I'm feeling very blessed these days. My wife, practice and well-being are all healthy and improving. What's more, I just received word my longtime dream has come true: the New York Museum of Modern Art selected one of my video games for exhibition. I am now a MoMA artist. OMG! When I created this game 30 years ago, I never imagined it would bring me here.

This did many things for me. One is to finally answer the long standing question: Are video games an art form? According to MoMA, yes they are! In the entertainment technology field we are very aware of the boundary between art and science; we just don't know where it is.

Why am I telling you? Because of a more recent question posed by one of my video game colleagues. He asked me: "Is psychotherapy an art or a science?" Hmmm. It's an interesting question, and one I'm giving some thought.

How much of what we do is actually scientifically based? Science is about repeatability, consistency and reducing variation. Science would dictate being the structured practitioner. But isn't the variation in life experience, situation, background and personal composition something to be utilized rather than minimized?

While chatting enjoyably with colleagues, I find Gut, Presence, Feel and Intuition are among the most frequently cited "effective" modalities in the room. These are tricky things to teach and regulate (standardize). Here lies the Art.

It's a classic conundrum, the tangible versus the ephemeral. Spontaneity on demand. Scheduling feelings. Science speaks to the body. Art speaks to the mind. Therapy must accommodate both.

Typically, when people want results they seek a scientist. Insurance companies rate various modalities against each other and the demand for Empirically Verifiable Therapy (EVT) seems to push the "therapy as science" stance. Providers must conform to scientific standards of repeatability, formatted reporting and consistency of practice. This argument is not without merit. It carries the weight of a major source of compensation for many therapists. There is also the educational benefit since it's easier to train scientists than artists. It also addresses the idea of getting the most care to the most people, just not tailoring the experience on an individual basis.

But what is the real cost of moving toward EVT? By reducing our flexibility are we lowering the level of care we provide? Are we losing the high end of what practice can be by moving toward a standardized version of therapeutic practice to get blessed by insurance carriers and the health care bureaucracy? Or are we just creating different market segments and new opportunities?

It has long been acknowledged that many modes of therapy cannot be studied empirically. Are we creating a world in which the only valid modes of therapy are the ones we can study?

In an attempt to answer one question I wound up with many. Here's another:

It seems to me the more we focus on standardizing the process the more we remove the human factor, the you-me-here-now component. If we believe the research which states rapport and client connection are the *most significant* determinants of positive outcomes then aren't we stepping away from best practices by moving toward standardization?

It's possible the issue of Art vs. Science gets confused along the same lines as Process vs. Content. Asking if something is an Art or a Science may be inviting ourselves to get stuck in content. Art and Science can be styles of approach and simply treatment possibilities rather than absolutes. They may be processes for therapy and may coexist comfortably (and in our therapeutic heart of hearts, I believe they frequently do).

Art or Science? The truth is usually in the middle so let's call therapy a Medium. A medium which allows for the expression of both Art and Science. This leaves practitioners a larger field with the freedom to choose the best approach for each client. For me, this is a very happy medium.

WHAT IS IT?

Here is another Fundamental Question of Personality:

It is what it is OR it isn't what it should be?

Which way do you sway when something you'd prefer wasn't, is?

It-is-what-it-is types lean more toward acceptance, seeking attunement with their environment. They tend to find more peace and derive energy from the environment. Their impact is more subtle and they are less inclined to demand change around them.

It-isn't-what-it-should-be types lean more toward judgment, seeking conformity to expectations. They tend to find less peace and infuse energy into the environment. Their impact is more overt and they are less inclined to leave things as they are.

Both are necessary, neither is sufficient. We are each capable of either and may shift between them from moment to moment. Together they form a Yin/Yang of personality.

I believe the world is both created and destroyed by it-isn't-what-it-should-be moments.

I also believe it-is-what-it-is moments make the world a more satisfying place to be.

The question remains: How can I balance the two?

Passion ☯ Perspective

"It is hard to love someone when you need them to change."

Maria Klein, MFT

"True strength is the ability to be appropriate in the moment."

Carolyn Kananen, MFT

THIS CANNOT BE BORING

I believe it is inaccurate to say "That's boring." Boredom is not an inherent property of any object or experience.

The accurate statement is "I'm bored by this," or "I find this boring." Boredom is something we bring to the party.

If the thing itself was inherently boring then every single person to encounter it would find it boring and I don't think anything like that exists.

What's more, when we say "that's boring," we are abdicating responsibility for how we feel. It's like blaming the sun for being warm. I may not like warm temperatures, but that's not the fault of the climate.

Every time I find a way to hold something else responsible for how I feel, I'm taking a step away from myself… and in doing so I'm reducing my possibilities for improving the situation.

Imagine a situation in which you're unsatisfied yet unable to do anything about it. Wouldn't you find that boring?

THE "SIGH" IN PSYMART

Happy New Year! I hope your holidays were joyous. My scale (and my wardrobe) are intimating I overindulged a tad this season. The only real casualty being the alterations I had done in November. Oh well, as you sew so shall you rip. But it's all good. A new year's in the offing. So full of hope and possibility. A fresh opportunity… to go to PsyMart, the one-stop shopping haven for therapists.

As I enter I see the ceiling girders are alive with brightly colored banners rhythmically swaying in the incense-laden breeze. They promise new groups, new marketing plans, new commitments. I love New Years at PsyMart!

But alas, today is not about the usual reverie and abandon, I'm here to make a return. A valued colleague gave me one of those clever calendars, unfortunately it's missing the months of May and July. My year goes by too fast as it is. I'm determined to recoup this tragic loss.

A PsyMart Customer Experience Facilitator approaches and asks: "How may I enhance your presence in this moment?"

"This moment is perfect… but this calendar is defective and I'd like to return it. Where can I go?"

"That depends on your priorities. For complaints I'd recommend Victim Validation, section B-9. But to move toward resolution you'll want the Unfinished Business Department. They're located in the kiosk by the food court until their offices are completed."

Unfinished Business it is. I start strolling across the endless sea of aisles that is PsyMart. Along the way, a video monitor catches my eye. They're touting "The Jung & The Restless," a new reality show about psychoanalysts in a sleep disorder clinic. It might be fun but it sounds like a thinly veiled remake of Generalized Hospital.

As I'm approaching the food court an intern hands me a coupon which reads: "Kentucky Freud Chicken - Electra-fying Deal! 50% off any Combo at our Transference Counter." I ask the intern if it's any good? "Absolutely!" she says, "I've eaten there 3 times-a-week for years and I'm still going."

I thank her for her input and start to walk on when I can't help overhearing a customer at the Reframing Window, "I get extremely upset when I tell my dog to stay and he doesn't listen."

"Try changing the dog's name to *Nama*."

"How will that help?"

"He may still disobey, but you'll be reminded to honor your own inner peace each time you say… '*Nama, Stay!*'"

PsyMart has an interesting take on service provision.

At last, the kiosk is in sight. As I cross the food court I contemplate the notion of fast food for therapists. Is it really a brief modality? There's Kentucky Freud Chicken, right between the Hungry HIPAA and my personal favorite, the Department of Consuming Éclairs. But this is no time for distractions.

At the kiosk sits a woman of great composure, and several empty chairs. There is no sign indicating the Unfinished Business Department, but the "UB" on her PsyMart uniform is all the confirmation I need. Her face neither smiles nor frowns, yet it invites me to speak.

"This calendar is missing two months. I want a complete one."

"OK, but first please take a moment to be the calendar. Describe your experience as the calendar."

"I'm not whole. I'm paginated and incomplete. I feel pressured. I feel a need to make up for lost time."

"Speak to me as the calendar. What does the calendar say?"

"I want a refund."

"Your experience cannot be refunded. The past is gone, we can only assist you with baggage. Speak to me as the baggage you carry from this calendriacal trauma."

"How about a store credit?"

"Excellent. Now *be* the store credit. Speak to the calendar…"

Two hours later I got a store credit, and a tremendous sense of well being.

Whether the giver or the givee, service can be challenging. However, when I allow myself to simply be curious and explore, PsyMart becomes an amazing place. I'm devoting this year to quality time in service. In fact, I'm putting it on my calendar.

Happy New Year!

A CONVENIENT TRUTH

You are OK right now. Whatever is going on, you are OK.

I'm not saying everything in your life is OK. I'm just saying that you, fundamentally, are OK.

You may not feel OK. You may think you cannot be OK until some future ambition is realized (graduation, promotion, financial status), but that is not the truth. The truth is you are OK right now.

Holding on to this idea that you can't be OK until later has serious implications…

It means one of the most fundamental aspects of your security and sense-of-self is unavailable for the foreseeable future. It means you are waiting on some unsure future condition to establish your well-being.

It means you don't exist right now.

Is that anything to feel anxious or panic about? You bet it is!

Fortunately, you really are OK right now. You have only to realize and accept it.

Passion ☯ Perspective

Parents who dine on the gratitude
of their children frequently go
to bed hungry.

The difference between self-aware-ness
and self-consciousness may be self-
judgment.

FAILURE'S VALUE

Failure is not an end, it's a launching point.

How do I know? I created the E.T. video game for Atari, one of the epic fails of our time. A failure so huge, Hollywood actually made a movie about it! Here's what I learned:

Failures are stepping stones to success... but only if we learn from them. Fail big! Fail boldly!!! But try to make each failure only once.

As Sherlock Holmes told Watson, "When you have eliminated the impossible, whatever remains, however improbable, must be the truth." So it is with success.

As you pursue various goals in life, the probability of succeeding increases with every failure found and passed... so long as you pay attention, keep learning and keep going.

I believe every action inherently contains both success and failure. One of the biggest questions in life is: Can you find them?

Always true => You've succeeded in arriving here now.

Always true => You've failed to be anywhere else.

This is more than optimism vs. pessimism. It's about gleaning the value from each, learning the lessons they conceal. Therein lies the greatest power in life.

NEW YEAR'S RESOLVED

How are your New Year's resolutions going?

I had big plans at the outset of this year. There were new marketing approaches, practice-enhancing ideas, writing projects and a few new tricks to apply in the room. Feeling tremendously excited about the coming year I was poised to hit the ground running…

Unfortunately, the ground hit me first. A few days after Christmas I developed a massive cold which evolved into a lingering hacking cough. I probably caught it during my last visit to PsyMart. It lasted for weeks and put an 'or' right in the middle of everything, turning my expectations into expect-or-ations, yuck!

What a bummer! I had planned to start the year at the top of my game, not under the weather. By the time I was fully reconstituted one thing was clear: My hotly anticipated pristine year of promise and potential was already slipping away. I was given to a bit of brooding over this sad state of affairs, finding myself weeks behind schedule in a year barely weeks old. What's up with that? And by "that" I mean the brooding! If a client told me this story I'd have two (optionally hyphenated) words for them: Self Care!!! It's time to do the work. Therapist, heal thyself!

Clearly my first important act of the year has to be forgiveness. I advise myself to accept my health situation, reset my calendar and get back into a positive mindset. But the weight of lost time and possibilities nags at me. Shouldn't I be getting more done? Can't I use my downtime more effectively? I keep coming up short in my year-to-date progress assessment. This is not exactly the kind of forgiveness I had in mind. So, I redirect my mind to pay more attention to what is happening, here's what I notice:

I find when I make resolutions about stopping this or doing more of that, I'm either succeeding or failing with every decision and I'm constantly judging myself. It occurred to me this is a messed-up way to begin a year. Then some real self-care kicked in!

I decide to call a do-over. Resetting my calendar is not enough. I need to reset my New Year's intention and chose a new style of resolution. I'm applying the formula: To transform anxiety into joy, simply transform "I have to" into "I get to." Instead of making my typical *demand-resolutions* about things I must do, I'm switching to *resolutions of opportunity* which are more about ways I may aspire to be. Here's how this works…

Instead of picking a task to execute or a restriction to abide, I choose how I might like to experience the year. What kinds of feelings, insights or directions might highlight such a year? Once that's settled, I resolve to find and engage those opportunities as they arise. As an example, here's my new New Year's resolution format:

I declare this to be The Year of Inspiration & Innovation.

Consequently, my resolution is to find inspiration wherever I can and be more inspiring to others. I would like to improve my effectiveness as well, so I'm going to pay more attention to others in hopes of learning new (and potentially more productive or gratifying) ways of doing things. I can't always plan how I'll do it, but I'll know when it's happening and I'll enjoy those moments.

It's easier to ratify an intention occasionally than to stay in a box constantly. I have goals too, and I'm working on them. But that's different, goals are not resolutions.

When I make resolutions about aspiring to potential, it's great when it happens and every little bit counts. If it's not happening I'm still open and present for the next opportunity. It's a more positive approach and that's how I prefer to engage my year.

It's never too late to resolve a Happy New Year!

CHOOSING POWER

"Life isn't about finding yourself. Life is about creating yourself." George Bernard Shaw

The very earliest parts of life are about discovering ourselves as a distinct part of the world, like in a movie when the image starts way out of focus then slowly becomes sharper and sharper until everything is clear. That's the beginning, figuring out what is.

But it doesn't take too long to get there. When I do, I gain the opportunity to shift from "figuring out what is" to "deciding what will be." Now the journey is about creating and manifesting. Taking my destiny into my own hands.

That's a big responsibility, but it is also an awesome gift! This is the point where my choices become incredibly important. Now I have the power to choose my own path.

I can choose to open and expand my possibilities or constrict them. I can choose to follow my own compass or meet the expectations of others.

Considering the potential of a human life, this is a lot of power indeed!

Passion ☯ Perspective

"Therapy is guiding people inside
themselves in ways that produce
new material."

Rob Fisher, MFT

"Our goal is not to be right;
our goal is for our clients
to experience themselves."

Maria Klein, MFT

ALWAYS REMEMBER...

On a surface level you face a seemingly endless parade of pitfalls and annoyances that nip at your heels and invite you into resistance and discomfort. Do not RSVP!

Know that on a deeper level you are undertaking a heroic journey to become someone who authentically devotes their life to improving the world by soothing distress while increasing joy, acceptance and hope. You are not your paperwork, reading list and schedule. You are a healer in heart and spirit, soon to be validated in credential. You are walking a noble path. This is who you are and you prove it every day you go to work!

Your courage and commitment inspire me, may it do the same for you.

DEFINED AT LAST

What is therapy? I keep coming back to this question. Therapy can be a first step, a second chance or a last resort.

I see therapy as an opportunity for growth. Genuine growth always creates change.

A therapist is a bridge between what is and what could be. Therapy is the journey from the outlook that's keeping you stuck to new perspectives that free you. Therapy is a journey of reexamining attitudes, leading to shifting perceptions and patterns.

Releasing attachment to outcomes is a very important part of this journey. This may seem counter-intuitive. After all, isn't the outcome the whole reason I come to therapy! What would I seek if not outcomes?

How about growth? Consider this: When we commit to specific outcomes we are limited. When we commit to growth we are free.

Grow your perspective in new directions. The more you expand your possibilities the more your outcomes will improve! Everyone is the genius of their own perspective. Be the best genius you can be!

I recently attended an excellent training given by Rob Fisher. One of the highlights for me was when Rob gave a definition of therapy. He said something along the lines of:

Therapy is guiding people inside themselves in ways that produce new material.

What an elegant description! How often do we reconsider long standing issues only to come up with the same old stuff? A good therapist helps you find new answers to old questions. Now you can explore new possibilities, pursue new directions and ultimately live a life of your own creation. A life better suited to who you are.

When I asked Rob for the exact quote I discovered another point about therapy...

He couldn't repeat the exact quote. The insight came to him in the moment, he shared it and then released it. I felt the impact and I carry the benefit forward, but the moment was gone and so were the particulars of the quote.

People who are truly present and focused in the moment produce remarkable things, but it can be hard to recall them later because the same focus that produced those gems has moved on to new moments. That's why recording can be a valuable tool.

Therapy happens in the present moment. The past is important, but nothing is ever solved or resolved there. The only place growth and healing occur is right here, right now.

Therapy is extremely spontaneous.

And what of the job of the therapist?

To paraphrase Albert Einstein, "We cannot solve our problems with the same thinking that created them."

People rarely come to a therapist to remain where they are. They want to fix, alter, manage, improve, adapt to and/or extricate themselves from some situation that currently occupies too much of their attention in some less than fabulous way. In short, they come to a therapist to make a change.

If we believe Einstein, then truly changing our circumstance requires changing our point of view. After all, tunnel vision only leads farther down the tunnel.

There are many ways to describe the job of a psychotherapist, and many ways to do that job. One way to view therapy is determining how others understand the world and ascertaining how I might expand or open them to new options and directions. What a fascinating and challenging task!

Toward this end I perpetually strive to find new ways to conceptualize and/or experience things. The broader my experiential base, the better I might meet each client's specific needs. It's not about telling people what to do. It's about creating moments which allow clients to discover for themselves what they want, thus creating the option of pursuing it.

If I tell you how a flower smells can you savor the fragrance? No. But if I can help you find some flowers, you can sample them for yourself. Now your life experience is genuinely richer and you have a larger base from which to proceed. Where you go from there is up to you.

ABOUT THE AUTHOR

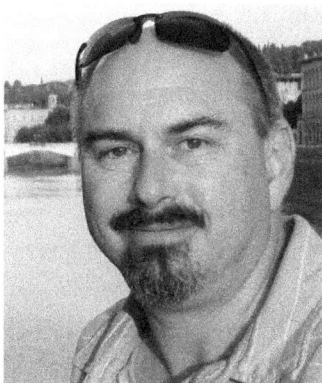

Howard Scott Warshaw holds degrees in Counseling Psychology, Computer Engineering, Economics, Mathematics and Theatrical Production. He is a MoMA artist as well as a celebrated pioneer of the video game industry. During his time in Silicon Valley he's published books and articles, programmed industrial robots and directed award winning documentary films.

Howard is many things to many people, but he is first and foremost a communicator. He is always looking for fresh perspectives to share with others.

Howard loves practicing psychotherapy because it utilizes every aspect of his eclectic skill set in the service of others. His private practice in Los Altos, CA focuses on the unique needs of individuals and couples in Silicon Valley's Hi-Tech community. Howard is also dedicated to cultivating and guiding MFT trainees and interns on their journey to licensure.

Find Howard (and his blog) at www.hswarshaw.com.

If you enjoyed this book, you may also want to read:

"Conquering College: *The most fun you can have learning the things you need to know*" available now on Kindle through Amazon.

This book teaches Howard's system for maxing college performance, minimizing work and saving up to one full year's tuition which he did while working on his Bachelor's degree.

BOOK PREVIEW: ONCE UPON ATARI

Here are the first two chapters of my upcoming book about Atari and the impact Atari has had on my life. Especially as it relates to the E.T. video game and the crash of the industry.

It's an autobiographical jaunt from my earliest years all the way through the Alamogordo dig. I originally planned to finish the book in 2019, but it should be done by the summer of 2020. It's taking more time to write than I had planned for two good reasons:

First, the project has gotten bigger, deeper and better along the way, and I believe there's no benefit to ignoring improvements as they present themselves.

Second, and more importantly, I refuse to make the same mistake with the book about the ET video game that I did with the game itself. Specifically, I'm not going to let a schedule determine the quality of the work! Instead, I'm allowing the quality of the work to determine the schedule.

Check out these first two chapters and see if this feels like it's going to be a level of quality worth waiting for…

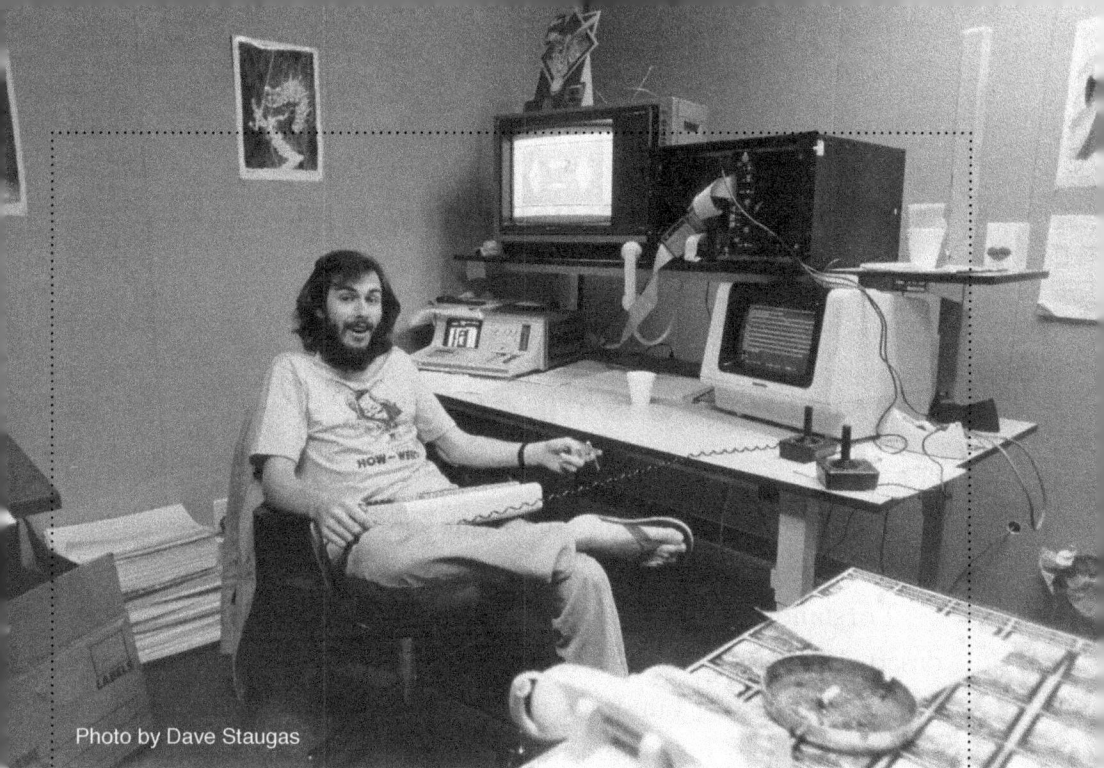
Photo by Dave Staugas

Once Upon ATARI

HOW I MADE HISTORY BY KILLING AN INDUSTRY

By Howard Scott Warshaw

CHAPTER 1:
LIGHTNING STRIKES

THE STORM BEFORE THE CALM

"Ouch!"

Airborne grains of sand and flying bits of old trash are pelting me without mercy. Honestly, I never imagined I'd find myself here...

I'm standing in the middle of a garbage dump in the New Mexico desert. It's hot. It's LOUD. A huge sandstorm rages all around us. I'm surrounded by hundreds of people from all over the country. We huddle like penguins for protection against the onslaught. There are news people, construction people, food people, film people and even some local politicians, but the vast majority are fans. Classic Video Game fans. People who smile at the mere mention of the word "Atari." They smile because this word summons deeply cherished memories.

We're all here, braving the heat and the storm, watching huge noisy yellow machines reaching deep into the ground, literally digging up my past right before my eyes. A big yellow arm disappears into a hole, bringing up another claw-bucket of ancient garbage and detritus. The arm swings around and dumps its load before returning for the next scoop, leaving behind a dusty pile of garbage. The ground between the machines and a thin plastic retaining fence is dotted with such piles. Each one holds the promise of a "nugget." Bodies press against the fence, straining to get a closer look at the latest droppings. "Is it there?" "Can you see one?" Or is this just more ammunition for the relentless gusting winds.

What are we doing here? We're searching for evidence. Specifically, we're hoping to unearth the murder weapon with which

I allegedly killed a multibillion-dollar industry back in the early '80s. And as good suspects do, I'm denying its existence. For decades I've said the very idea is ridiculous, but today I really hope I'm wrong. I've explained many times over why this whole operation makes absolutely no sense. But I'd forgotten the cardinal rule:

When you expect things to make sense, you're losing touch with Atari.

This is another remarkable day in my life. I've had many, but this one is special. Saturday, April 26th, 2014 is the longest day of my life, because it started on July 27th, 1982.

THE PHONE CALL

On the afternoon of Tuesday, July 27th, 1982 I'm sitting in my office at 275 Gibraltar Drive, Atari's headquarters in Sunnyvale, California. I'm hanging out with Jerome Domurat after putting the final touches on Raiders of the Lost Ark, the longest development of all my games. Jerome is my graphics/animation designer as well as my good friend. We're having fun in our usual way, taking turns reading aloud from National Lampoon magazine's letters to the editor, when a call comes in: "Will you please hold for Ray Kassar?"

Will I hold for Ray Kassar? The Chief Executive Officer of Atari? My boss's boss's boss's boss's boss? The guy who signs my checks? "Yes, I'll hold for him."

A phone call from Ray Kassar is a very unusual thing in my experience. However, this is not my first time chatting enjoyably with our CEO. The first time was at a press event. I was demo-playing my first game, Yars Revenge, on one of the first ever Big-Screen TVs (a hulking rear-projection monstrosity). Ray emerged from the slew of media people crawling around the room. He approached me and said, "Hello Howard, I heard about what you did with Yars."

"Yeah? What did you think about that, Ray?"

He half-smiled, "Just keep making games, Howard." Then he turned and melted back into the traffic. That was my first encounter with Ray Kassar. The last time we met, however, was a bit more memorable…

Roughly two months before answering this phone call, I was nearing the final stages of development on Raiders of the Lost Ark, the first ever video game based on a movie. It was a dog-and-pony day, which means some key execs would cruise engineering for demos (somewhat akin to visiting the zoo). We would show the current state of our games to anyone being escorted by our bosses. I took game demos pretty seriously, but today was special. Ray Kassar was coming down from on high to take the tour himself, and he had quite an entourage. Several extras, including marketing, legal and the odd vice president. You know it's Ray coming because his distinctive cologne always precedes him. He came wafting in and took the guest chair while the others stood around him like a halo of nodding assent. I had the game ready to go and Tchaikovsky's "Overture of 1812" (the one with the cannons) cued up on the office stereo. It lends an impressive ambiance to the demonstration, well beyond the capabilities of my development station.

[NOTE to the Non-Nerd: A Development Station (or Dev Station) is a specialized piece of hi/low-tech computer hardware (frequently tucked into a black metal box) where game programmers can test-run and debug their software in a reliable environment. It is designed to prevent programmers from having anything other than themselves to blame for their product issues. Of course, this design goal is not always realized.]

I press Play on the stereo, pick up my game controller and roll through the demo.

Ray would make a comment here and there which was quickly and enthusiastically affirmed by the entourage.

Now it isn't every day I get Ray Kassar in my office, so being the braying ass I'm given to be at times like this in my mid 20's, I took the opportunity to share some thoughts and suggestions (read: criticisms & complaints) as to how the company might be better run. Mouthing off to the big man is not usually the smartest strategy, but it's easier when your work represents a significant chunk of corporate profits, past and future.

After sitting politely through a more-than-reasonable bit of this, Ray cuts in and says, "Interesting ideas. Perhaps we should switch jobs for a day."

Instantly I fire back, "I'm good with that, Ray. Here's my dev station. Just give me your fragrance and let's go."

And the room froze.

Uh-oh. Have I gone too far this time? (a question I ask myself all too frequently)

A deafening silence hung there, occasionally broken by stifled chortles. The entourage wants to laugh but they don't want the guillotine. All the king's men were desperately trying to hold their laughter until they got some inkling of Ray's reaction. After what seemed like hours, Ray decided to find it amusing and thus unleashed the torrent. Laughter abounded as they shuffled on to the next office.

Since I wasn't fired for that one, I lived to take this call...

Ray comes on the phone and gets right to the point: "Howard, we need an E.T. game for September 1st. Can you do it?"

Without missing a beat, I say, "Absolutely I can! Provided we reach the right agreement." I know what I mean. Ray knows too. Money.

"That's fine," Ray says, "be at San Jose Airport Thursday morning at 8am. There will be a Learjet waiting to take you to Spielberg's office where you'll present the design for the game."

And there it is. I'm doing the E.T. game! My first thought is: Whoa, I've got 36 hours to do the entire design and prepare a presentation for the fastest video game development ever attempted. My second thought is: Better have a good dinner tonight, it might need to last me a while. And oh yeah, I'm still on the phone…

I assure Ray I'll be fully prepared when I board the Spielberg-express first thing Thursday morning. We say our goodbyes and hang up. This would not be my first encounter with Steven Spielberg. We'd met several times before, but this one will require more imagination, creativity and preparation than any other. It would also end up needing the kind of fancy footwork you can't practice in advance.

I know what I'm actually promising. Games on this system usually take at least 6 months to develop. I'm committing to do one in 5 *weeks*. Am I confident? My hubris is. But right now, I'm already too busy to think about it. Just 36 hours to my first delivery milestone. In order to pull this off, a lot of headwork needs to happen in a very short time. Fortunately, my brain is hard-wired for fast. The tricky part is the balance, staying focused but not tunnel visioned…

Let the thinking begin!

So… where to go for dinner?

CHAPTER 2:
KING LEARJET

BACK TO THE DESERT

And now we're back in the New Mexico desert in 2014, because this isn't just a chronicle, it's also a time machine. And a good thing too, because it takes a time machine to understand how that one phone call decades ago began paving a road leading me to this place, this hour, this sandstorm in a dump in the desert.

Today started several hours earlier and nearly 5,000 feet higher in a mountaintop hideaway hotel, far from this chaos. After a hearty breakfast, we boarded the van of destiny and headed for the Alamogordo city dump. Winding our way down snaking mountain roads, I was feeling both curious and anxious. Curious about what they'd find under the ground and anxious about what that might mean. Upon arrival, I see something very odd indeed... there's a line of people waiting. A long line. When's the last time you saw hundreds of people standing in line to get into a garbage dump?

I should probably say a bit more about what's going on here. Today, Lightbox & Fuel Entertainment (Hollywood production companies), Xbox Entertainment Studios (a small part of a *huge* corporate entity) and the city of Alamogordo, New Mexico are jointly hosting (and filming) a modern archeological event. This is an excavation (or "dig") to literally uncover the truth behind an enduring urban myth. Specifically, that decades ago Atari trucked millions of unsold E.T. video game cartridges into the desert and buried them here in this dump. I'm here too of course, because I did it. I'm the one.

I made the worst video game of all time!

139

This is not my opinion. This is the conclusion held by many All-Time lists. Go ahead, Google "worst video games of all time" and see what you get. Countless fans and media people remind me of this "fact" regularly. In 1995, New Media magazine said my E.T. game was so bad it single-handedly caused the video game crash of the early '80s, collapsing an industry with revenues approaching four billion dollars.

It was so bad that Atari needed to bury it way out in the desert just to get rid of the stench! At least that's the legend. Snopes.com says it's true. I don't think so. I've always denied it. I'll tell you why...

When a company is hemorrhaging money to the tune of hundreds of millions of dollars and they find themselves sitting on a mountain of worthless inventory, why would they spend even more money to transport, crush, cement over and bury that inventory? That's a very expensive thing to do. Why not recycle the materials to reduce the cost of making new product that might sell? At the very least, you could simply throw open the doors of the warehouse and let people come in and take it all. Why spend big money getting rid of something you believe is worthless? It doesn't make any sense.

As I said before, when you expect things to make sense, you're losing touch with Atari.

Atari was never about making sense. Atari was about making fun. It was about inventing things that never existed before in ways no one had ever done. It was not a sensible place; it was an outrageous place. It was an orgy of creativity and innovation, populated by the most engaging, accomplished and eccentric cast of characters I've ever known. Atari was the perfect place at the perfect time for me... but they didn't see it at first.

After a round of interviews Atari rejected me... but it didn't stick. I pushed back. I reasoned, argued, and pleaded with Dennis Koble (the hiring manager running my interview process) until he finally agreed to give me a chance (for a probationary period and a significantly smaller salary)(which I gladly accepted). I kept pushing, because on some deep intuitive level I knew Atari would be my home. It was everything I needed for sustenance and growth in my life. I had to be there… and I had to belong there.

When my time at Atari ended (which it had to, since nothing so imbalanced can remain standing indefinitely) I knew it would never be equaled. And it never was.

I did finally exceed it, however. After some thirty years of searching, schooling & internships I finally became what I always wanted to be: a psychotherapist. And now, with my life once again supremely satisfying and rewarding, I find myself in the desert getting sandblasted at the end of a long and winding road which began decades ago with a phone call. I'm waiting to see if my past will rise once more. Is my notorious creation poised to jump out of this ever-deepening hole in the desert floor?

I hope it does, it'll make for a much better movie that way. In fact, the prospect of being wrong has never been more appealing. Besides, I always want my games to be groundbreaking in some fashion. Will my third creation finally break ground in a new and most unexpected way? The irony would be delicious. Speaking of which, I'm getting kind of hungry…

YOUR LEARJET AWAITS

I hate getting up early in the morning. Aside from a brief stint in commercial real estate, I've always worked hard to maintain a life that never needs an alarm clock. It's just no way to start the day. However, when a Learjet is waiting to take you to Steven Spielberg's office, it eases the sting considerably.

I make it to the airport at the appointed hour and there, to my considerable delight, is an actual Learjet waiting just for me. Guess what? I love airports and airplanes! Took my first flight at two weeks old and I've enjoyed it ever since. In this moment, I'm incredibly psyched. This promises to be another remarkable day in my life.

I board the jet and take the first of the 6 seats. The pilot is kind enough to leave the cabin door open (it is 1982, after all). I can see right through the cockpit windows without having to move from my incredibly comfy chair. I ease back and wait for the show to begin. The takeoff is smooth and soon we are soaring just above the clouds. It's always amazing to see the sea of clouds, so soft, serene and endless. It seems such a beautiful place to stroll, but I decide to remain in my seat just the same. We're flying to Burbank, and then on to Warner Studios where Spielberg and his sprawling office await. But it turns out we're not going to Burbank, at least not yet. First, we'll stop in Monterey to pick up some additional passengers.

As we near the Monterey area, a most unsettling sight appears through the pilot's windshield. The usual soft white carpet of clouds is now punctuated with a cluster of mountain tops. As we descend through the bright white layer and the visibility shrinks to zero, I can't help thinking that mountain tops usually have mountains underneath them. In this case, I'm really hoping I'm wrong.

Fortunately, the pilot missed every single one of them and landed cleanly on the Monterey runway. He taxied a bit, then came to rest on a vacant section of tarmac. Nearly vacant that is, because just as the plane slowed to a stop a big black limo pulls up right off the left wing. The doors open and out pops Ray Kassar (CEO), Skip Paul (Chief Legal Counsel) and Lyle Rains (Coin-Op Game Engineer). Apparently, Lyle is doing the arcade version of E.T., and I'll bet he's getting more than 5 weeks too! OK, I didn't really think this last part. After all, this is only 40 hours into the project so I'm not bitter yet. As they file onto the plane, I hear Skip say to Ray, "What? They couldn't get the Hawker?!" He sounds disappointed, but this is hard for me to imagine. They take their seats and away we go. The takeoff is carefree since mountains aren't nearly so scary on this side of the clouds.

We fly for a while more, Ray and Skip are chatting a bit but Lyle and I are silent. The time of the presentation is approaching, this means the tension and the focus is building. We land in Burbank airport and once again, just as the plane comes to a halt another limo pulls up alongside. "It's just like in the movies," I think to myself, but I guess it makes sense since we're going to meet Steven Spielberg at Warner Studios. This is so cool, I can hardly believe it's a workday… but it is, which makes it even cooler. I'm loving this.

We get in the limo, and it's a remarkably well-appointed vehicle. In addition to the plush seating accommodations, there is a phone, a TV, a small fridge and even a sink. Skip reaches over and pushes the lever to watch the water stream out, but nothing happens. The amazing thing was the look on his face. He says, "Do you believe it, the water doesn't even work." OMG! He's serious. This guy just got off a private jet into a waiting limo and he's actually annoyed that the water isn't running in the car's sink. I realize we're from different worlds, and much as I'd like to belong, I'm not really a part of his. I'm always interested to get a glimpse into other people's perspectives. Not always relieved, but definitely interested.

The guard waves us through the gate at Warner and we proceed along the lot until we arrive at the office. We go in and pleasantries are exchanged all around. Now it's presentation time and Lyle goes first, which gives me a little time to chill. My thoughts begin to drift. Spielberg's office is small… for a luxury apartment. It's nice to be back here again. A calm settles in… but not for long. "Wait a minute," I think to myself, "why am I here?"

It occurs to me I don't have an answer. I realize it's because I said "yes" of course, but why did Ray call me directly? That's never happened before. This has all been so exciting, I forgot how odd it was. Atari is big on secret culture and back channel communications, there is always something going on you don't know about. Here's what I didn't know:

I was not the first person Ray called about doing the E.T. game. His first call was to George Kiss, my grandboss (or boss's boss). George is the head of engineering for the Atari home game system, and he told Ray what any sane and knowledgeable person in that situation would: You cannot do a game in 5 weeks. It's simply not enough time. Case closed.

Most CEOs do not like "no" as an answer. It rarely contributes to shipping product and making money. So, after being told by the head of development it couldn't happen, Ray still thought it was worthwhile to make one more call. That's the value of relationships at work. I'd apparently built enough of a reputation or made enough of an impression that he believed I might come through when others couldn't. Or it might have to do with the time Ray saw my personal notebook and asked to peruse it. I lent it to him, and it came back through interoffice mail a few days later with a note attached. "Thank you, Howard. You are a Renaissance man." This is the nicest thing anyone can say to me.

This was all very flattering and, as I think about it now, rather creepy. I told Ray it absolutely would happen right after my grandboss told him it couldn't. Talk about undermining relationships. That's what I didn't know at the time, and I'm glad I didn't.

Suddenly, the question, "Howard, what have you got for us?" pierces my reverie and brings me back to the moment. Now it's my turn and I begin my presentation…

The last time I presented something to Spielberg was early June, about a month and a half ago. We met at the Consumer Electronics Show in Chicago and I had *the tape*. I was nearing completion on the Raiders of the Lost Ark game, my second project for Atari and my first for Spielberg. Atari needed a way to demonstrate the game for Spielberg in Chicago. I could have simply played it for him, but I thought it would be better to make a demo tape that could serve other promotional purposes as well. The execs agreed and sent me to a video recording studio to make the demo.

Have you ever done something absolutely perfectly? At exactly the right time? I did. Just once. At that studio.

They sat me down, put a mic on me, hooked up the console to a recorder and I played and narrated the entire game flawlessly. That had never happened in any of my demos, before or since. It was a magical moment. A one-take wonder. We added a few special effects, created a master and that was it. By the way, the total running time of that tape was 12 minutes and 27 seconds. If it takes you longer than this to play all the way through Raiders, you probably didn't make the game.

From the time I left that studio in Sunnyvale until this meeting in Chicago, the tape never left my side. There was NO WAY I was going to miss seeing Spielberg's reaction.

Full disclosure: I'm a huge film buff, and Steven Spielberg is a hero of mine. I love his work, from "Duel" on. I think Raiders of the Lost Ark is a masterwork and I was honored to be a part of it in this way. But I'm not just meeting my hero, I'm working with/for him. It's one thing to meet your idol, it's another to have them evaluate your work. It's another still when they evaluate your work which is a derivative of their work. This is huge for me... as long as he likes it.

For a serious creative person, a lot of self-image (and mental well-being) is on the line at a time like this. I was confident but very nervous. I'm one of the top video game creators of my time, but what I really want to be is a film director.

Finally, the moment came. There I was, up in the crow's nest of the enormous Atari show booth with a TV and a tape deck and Steven. I inserted the tape and hit PLAY. Spielberg watched it thoroughly and intently. He didn't move at all for the entire run time of 12 minutes and 27 seconds. I know because I watched him thoroughly and intently for the entire run time of 12 minutes and 27 seconds. At the end he thought for a bit, soaking it in. Then he looked up at me and said, "That's really great, Howard. It feels just like a movie!" My inner world exploded with joy. Steven Spielberg thinks the demo tape of my game for his movie feels like a movie... yeah BABY!

That was one of the greatest moments of my life... but that was then and this is now. I finish laying out the design for the E.T. game and Spielberg thinks for a bit, soaking it in. Then he looks up at me and says, "Couldn't you do something more like Pac-Man?"

My inner world collapses.

Something more like Pac-Man?!?! OMG! One of the most innovative film directors of all time wants me to make a knock off? My impulse is to say: "Gee Steven, couldn't you do something more like 'The Day The Earth Stood Still'?"

Fortunately, my brain kicks in microseconds before my mouth engages. Get a grip, Howard. This is Steven Spielberg, and he obviously likes Pac-Man. You were going to say it too, weren't you? My father's words came to me in this moment, he was fond of saying "Get your head out of your ass, wipe the shit from your eyes and focus!" Ah, the memories.

All this took a fraction of a second in my head. Then I regroup and take another tack entirely. "Steven, E.T. is amazing and we need something special to go with it. This is an innovative game for an innovative movie." I believe this is true, but I'm also aware of another fundamental truth: the game I'm proposing is one I might possibly *finish* in 5 weeks, a critical component of success in the overall delivery process.

That's why I need to defend this design with everything I've got. I'd rather not fall back on this explanation because I'd rather not come off as desperate, but I will if I must. It harkens back to one of the great linguistic contributions of computer science: Doability (noun, the quality of being able to be done. From the modern English; Do + Ability). Ask any software engineer about the prospect for a task or design, and the answer will invariably revolve around the word "doable." I'm confident this design has sufficient doability to be worth pursuing. This is distinct from another contribution: Bogosity (noun, the quality of being bogus, a mangle-ization of Bogus). Bogosity and doability are independent properties. In other words, creating a game in five weeks can have significant doability and still represent a high level of bogosity on the face of it. In other other words, the possibility of doing it doesn't make it a good idea. This paragraph stands as proof of this concept.

[NOTE to the Non-Nerd: Many people do not consider nerds to be facile linguists or communicators. Be advised: New-Word construction and deployment is an essential part of the nerd repertoire. To be clear, I'm talking specifically about techie nerds or geeks. Word nerds and/or grammar police are beyond the scope of this text.]

After a few moments of breath-holding, Steven relents on the Pac-Man proffer and accepts my assertion that the design is appropriate to the task at hand (the punishment fits the crime). As he does, I realize my design is now approved. Things are shaping up. The first major milestone is achieved, my inner world is resurrected, and (though I'm not 100% sure about this) there seems to be a faint emanation coming from Steven's chest, a sort of reddish glow. I have a theory about this...

But this is no time for theory. There are hard facts to face:

- An accepted design only opens the door to begin continuous crunch mode. It is truly the gift that keeps on taking.
- Tomorrow is day 4 of the 35.5 days allotted for the task, 10% of my schedule is already gone.
- I still have to make it through a Learjet ride home before I'm anywhere near dinner! (OK, not all the facts are hard)

I've got the design. It's implementation time. There's nothing to it but to do it!

And as the golden light of late afternoon kisses the flats and backlots of Warner studios, the Atari delegation boards the waiting limousine and sets off for the airport.

BOOK PREVIEW:
THE SILICON VALLEY THERAPIST

Here are some excerpts from a book I'm writing about the life and characters of Silicon Valley. As a former software developer/manager and a current psychotherapist, I spend much of my time helping the people who shape modern technology when their lives get out of shape.

This includes people at home with their relationships and people at work with their careers and job situations. I work with individuals and couples, as well as co-founders and key employees.

I address anything that might interfere with the personal or professional success of hi-tech leaders and the super-intelligent. It's quite interesting work because the denizens of Silicon Valley are a rather interesting bunch, and the conundrums they create for themselves, their co-workers and their loved ones are extraordinary to say the least.

But at the same time we are all human beings, dealing with the basic issues people have faced for thousands of years, we're simply doing it with newer tech these days...

YOU'RE NEVER TOO SMART
TO HAVE PROBLEMS
(DEBUNKING "INTELLIGENCE" MISCONCEPTIONS)

Intelligence is something we have many ideas about… and even more preconceptions. Some intelligent people believe their IQ absolves them of issues. Let me assure you, no one is too smart to have problems (though their complexes can be quite complex).

As The Silicon Valley Therapist, I help very intelligent people face real struggles resulting from the circumstances they were smart enough to get themselves into.

This may sound like a tough job, and it is at times. But the challenge isn't being more brilliant and solving their problems. The challenge is caring for and learning about them enough to guide them to their own solutions.

When working with the super-intelligent, I don't have to be smarter than my client to help them, I only need to be smart enough. Here are five points I've gleaned about intelligence which help me in this pursuit.

1. Intelligence is a Tool, not a Character Trait

Have you ever seen a smart person set out to (and fully succeed in) doing something stupid? Intelligence helps you achieve goals, it doesn't help you select them. Some goals solve problems and some goals create problems.

For any given task, a more intelligent person will likely complete it faster/better/cheaper than a less intelligent person. And when the goal is deceiving yourself? Well, intelligent people do that better too.

I'll bet that smarts, eh?

2. Intelligence Doesn't Define You, it Merely Enables You

Being intelligent doesn't make you right and it doesn't make you kind. Your knowledge base tends to determine rightness or wrongness, and your morality will likely determine the kindness in your heart.

Moral Character is a key aspect of how we define a person, and character exists completely independent of Intelligence. On the one hand we're either smart or simple, and on the other we can be good or bad. "He's not that bright but he's got a good heart" is a common expression of the simple/good combo. Movies teach us the most dangerous people come from the smart/bad hybrid. Super-heroes aren't challenged much by evil-dummy types. It takes an Evil Genius to make a blockbuster antagonist!

Who I am depends on my choices. Intelligence doesn't make the choices, it simply contributes to how I implement those choices.

3. Intelligence and Knowledge Are Two Separate Things...

...and they are not interchangeable. Knowledge is the data you've got; facts and details. Intelligence is your ability to use the data to achieve results. Greater intelligence creates more results with the same data.

This difference is quite notable when judging others (think: job interview). It is all too common for ignorance to be mistaken for low intelligence. This is unfortunate.

Ignorance is merely a lack of information which is easily countered by acquiring the information. Education cures ignorance. It's much harder to cure stupidity.

Of course, it's a lot easier to *test* knowledge than intelligence. When interviewers confuse knowledge with intelligence, their hiring decisions tend to suffer.

How many Einstein's are working the fields today? What is the price of overlooking some great brains? What key problems in the world might have been solved by now?

4. IQ and EQ Are Two Separate Things

IQ estimates our intelligence potential. EQ estimates our potential for relating emotionally with self and others. IQ tends to get more attention, but EQ is a far better predictor of success. Precious few endeavors in life are accomplished alone.

How we relate is a choice. Some people choose to use their brain power to separate themselves from others. They are Brain-Bullies. Brain-bullies strive to create the impression: "I'm smarter than you, and I'll prove it by running to places where you can't keep up with me."

If someone tries to beat me up with their "IQ", my best response is to lean on my EQ, for example…

Another way to hear the brain-bully is: "I'm scared out here in the open. I need to hide somewhere you can't reach me. Then maybe I'll feel safer." That's not being smart, that's just insecure.

When I view IQ through an EQ lens, people may shift from pathetic to sympathetic. Intelligence does not automatically create intellectual snobbery or pretension, that's just one option.

I believe a far better option is to use my intelligence to merge EQ & IQ. This means striving to make elusive concepts more accessible to others, not less. This increases the universal pool of knowledge and understanding, something which benefits everyone.

Pretense builds walls, Genius opens doors.

The choice is yours. By focusing more on EQ than IQ it becomes easier to be a smart person without being a jerk, and it also becomes easier to deal with a smart person without feeling jerked around.

5. The Logical End of Intelligence is Insanity

This is the flip side of Ignorance is Bliss.

The world can be a messed-up place, with seemingly endless examples of unnecessary suffering which could be addressed and alleviated… but aren't.

The smarter you are, the more frequently you may identify these situations. If you care, you would likely feel frustration and/or anguish. Over time, these feelings accumulate. It follows logically that carrying all this can become overwhelming and ultimately disabling.

Fortunately, people aren't entirely logical.

It's not mandatory to walk off the emotional cliff. But if we are to prevent becoming totally imbalanced there needs to be a path back towards balance. That path is Acceptance.

Accept that life's ugliness is balanced by beauty. Readjust your focus. Spend some time appreciating the wonder and delight which also abounds but is all too easily forgotten.

Accept the limits of your influence. Do what you can… but be realistic about your ability to alter circumstances (and other people).

Acceptance can be the difference between intelligence and insanity. It's the tool which lends perspective and activates life's primary shock absorber: Resiliency.

Armed with this information, it is my sincerest hope you will move forward in your life, better able to handle intelligence (both theirs and yours) more knowledgably!

FAILURE:

THE MISUNDERSTOOD GIFT

We enjoy our successes but we grow from our failures... or we don't.

The difference usually comes down to choices. I believe our experience of Failure speaks more to our choices than our circumstances.

What do I know about failure? Plenty.

I authored one of the greatest failures of my generation. I'm blamed for single-handedly destroying the billion-dollar video game industry of the early 1980's. I did this by creating the worst video game of all time: E.T. for the Atari 2600. A failure so huge, Hollywood actually made a movie about it! Check out "Atari: Game Over". And that's not even my greatest failure. I've been fortunate enough to have many, in all aspects of my life; personal, professional and relational.

From pioneering new tech to rewiring old habits, from real estate to filmmaking, from robotics to writing, my breadth of experience helps me understand the many ways things can go wrong and how best to deal with them.

I've had successes too, but I'm most grateful for my failures because they've enabled me to enlist my esoteric skillset in the service of healing a wider range of people. My failures have made me a better therapist... and a better person.

As The Silicon Valley Therapist, helping people deal with failure and disappointment is a core competency. Luckily, I've had lots of practice.

How does Failure fit into the fabric of your life?

Before you answer, please consider some lessons Failure taught me...

1. Failure is a Perspective, Not an Occurrence

Failure is not what happened. The happenings of life are neither successes nor failures, they are merely circumstances.

There are many possible interpretations we can put on those circumstances... Failure is only one of them. Our choices determine what we carry forward from the current situation, which then shapes how we handle our next encounter. When you mind what you bring to events, you bring a better mind to them.

2,000 years ago, Epictetus said "It is not events which shape our lives, but rather our view of the events." We choose how we view things, and these choices have far ranging life consequences.

Failure is a frame of mind, not a state of affairs.

2. Failure Lacks Context

So you failed. This may feel like hard times, but the truth is: It's impossible to know where you are until you see where it takes you. Life is complex and it's hard to predict how things will turn out from the current picture. The caterpillar and the butterfly share the same DNA.

This so-called failure is but a single moment in the story of your life. Why be so quick to judge your situation... or yourself?

After all, some failures turn out to be blessings in disguise. Have you ever invested yourself totally in winning a job/deal/accolade only to find out later it wasn't what you thought or hoped? Sometimes when I trip and fall, I wind up dodging a bullet.

It's also true that major failures are frequently enabled by significant successes. You can't fall too far unless you've first scaled the heights. Do you focus on the loss, or your ability to climb?

Every failure has the potential to launch you later. Early stumbles can be wakeup calls in disguise. This experience could be the greatest teacher you've ever had, please try to release your disappointment and zero in on the lesson.

Because…

3. Failure is a School, Not a Prison.

In life: Mistakes are mandatory, learning is optional.

The learning process can be seen as continually making mistakes and never repeating them. If I'm paying attention, I'm accumulating a pool of avoidable mishaps. Every failure has the potential to grow this pool, making each future "project" more likely to succeed.

But to implement this strategy I must be willing to review my failure and glean the lessons. What could stand in my way? Shame, fear and denial… exacerbated by ego.

Many are taught failure is bad. We may come to believe *we* are bad if we fail. Shame is an easy place to get stuck. Ego can lead me into denial and away from learning from my failures because ego can highlight my fears.

In the HiTech world, you can't swing a USB-cable without hitting a sizable ego. And denial runs rampant in many organizations (other people's denial is the easiest to spot). What we may not see so readily are the fear and shame lying beneath the surface.

Some fear failure so intensely they never try because they can't afford the risk. This is withdrawal, a self-limiting mindset.

Others are bolder. They're willing to try many things, but they are also ready to bend reality or rewrite history rather than face the shame of acknowledging any failed attempt. This is denial, and denial has a problem: While the denier denies the failure, the denial denies the denier the opportunity to learn from the failure.

Simply put, the price of denial is lost opportunity. This can be *very* expensive!

Locking yourself in the Prison of Shame & Denial is an option, but it isn't terribly productive. Punishing yourself for a miss doesn't do much to improve your aim next time around.

Why not punish less and learn more? Instead of judging yourself, go to school. Take the Failure Quiz:

What really happened here?
Did any of my actions help it go this way?
What might I change to improve my odds next time?

Answering these questions frankly and honestly results in a more robust toolbox…

4. Successfully Handling Failure Requires Tools

Here are two different worldviews:

Life is an unrelenting all-or-nothing make-or-break proposition where my wellbeing is constantly on the line.

-OR-

Life is a series of successive approximations in which I'm always learning and trying to do better next time.

Neither is guaranteed to be correct. You'll find super-achievers and ne'er-do-wells in both categories. Which feels more productive? Which better accommodates failure? Which one is currently you?

For my own part, I advocate the second, but I catch myself slipping into the first at times. When I do, it's my toolset which helps me get back on course.

The toolset for this second worldview consists of Curiosity, Resiliency, Humor and Forgiveness.

Curiosity is the single best tool for learning! Curiosity leads us to find value. Judging leads us to create drama and pain. Admitting and owning my failures requires honest self-assessment, not harsh self-judgment. Don't sell yourself short on shortcomings, they may be your greatest asset.

Resiliency is important as well, it's the shock absorber of life. When we get too fragile, even small bumps can break things. The easily shattered have a tough time moving into unpaved territory, which is where every next big thing comes from.

Humor is one of the greatest sources of resiliency. Laughing at my folly reduces its sting. For decades, people have asked me how it feels to have made the worst video game ever? I tell them I enjoy the distinction. I also made Yars' Revenge, frequently cited as one of the best games of all time. So if E.T. is the worst game ever, I have the *greatest range* of any game designer in history!

Humor is great medicine and it's always available. If you can't find the humor, you may be missing other things as well. Things that could help.

Forgiveness is another essential component. Forgiveness is not condoning or accepting transgressions, forgiveness is permitting myself not to spend today's energy on the indelible past which will never change. Energy wasted on resentment & regret is energy which could make the difference between success and failure on my current project. Forgiveness isn't something you give to another, it's a gift you give yourself.

Don't let failures become baggage. Own the fail, learn the lessons, then *let it go*. The more baggage you carry, the fewer doors you can fit through. Lighten your load and ease the journey.

5. The Big Win: Converting failure to wisdom!

Again: We enjoy our successes, but we *grow* from our failures… or we don't.

The way we grow is by converting our failures into wisdom which can guide us more effectively in future decisions. Failure is the #1 source of wisdom in life.

Think of Wisdom as a commodity. It's mined from the ore of our mistakes. Which means each of us is sitting on the mother lode! And like any mining operation, when the refinery is closed the stock price drops considerably.

In other words, every bit of wisdom you don't acquire makes you dumber than you would have been had you learned it. Don't worry, you're still just as smart as you are, you simply missed a chance to be smarter. Unfortunately, staying the same in a rapidly changing world means constantly losing ground. I need to make an occasional step forward just to stand still, so it's best to keep my refinery humming.

Therapy (like Life) is all about the breaks, breakdowns and breakthroughs. People come to me in the former and I help them find the latter. Know this: Time spent wallowing in the breakdowns is time that could be spent cultivating the breakthroughs. To paraphrase Einstein: You should move through it as fast as possible, but no faster.

Now that you have some new perspectives on Failure, consider this question:

How will Failure fit into the context of your life?

I believe it can be as simple as this: Life is a series of successive approximations. When I invest the effort to learn from my failures, my every "next step" is improved and my life's path converges on satisfaction and happiness.

When handled skillfully, Failure is not an end, it's a launching point!

NOTES

NOTES

www.ingramcontent.com/pod-product-compliance
Lightning Source LLC
Chambersburg PA
CBHW072135020426
42334CB00018B/1814